The Miracles of the Bible Viewed Differently

Maximilian Ledochowski

The Miracles of the Bible Viewed Differently

Part 1 the New Testament

Springer

Maximilian Ledochowski
Innsbruck, Austria

ISBN 978-3-031-51638-2 ISBN 978-3-031-51639-9 (eBook)
https://doi.org/10.1007/978-3-031-51639-9

Translation from the German language edition: "Die Wunder der Bibel medizinisch erklärt" by Maximilian Ledochowski, © Springer Nature 2023. Published by Springer Nature. All Rights Reserved.

This Springer imprint is published by the registered company Springer Nature Switzerland AG
The registered company address is: Gewerbestrasse 11, 6330 Cham, Switzerland

Paper in this product is recyclable.

Introduction

The New Testament describes numerous "miracles" that are meant to prove the "divinity" of Jesus and thus support the faith. Most of them are of a medical nature, miraculous healings, raising the dead and other occurrences that could not be explained with the knowledge of the time.

It is not possible to make medical diagnoses 2000 years after Christ lived. But if one interprets the symptoms described in the Bible with today's knowledge, diseases can be suspected or diagnoses can be assigned. Even today, many diagnoses are not only made with technical aids or blood tests, but only "clinically". This means that the doctor makes the diagnosis on the basis of the symptoms that the patient describes or on the basis of his observations. Thus, even today, the diagnosis of schizophrenia is not made by any laboratory tests, but on the basis of symptoms such as "descriptions of hallucinations", hearing commanding, so-called "imperative" voices or "dialogues with non-existent persons, so-called dialogizing voices", etc. So if someone in the Bible said that he heard the voice of God commanding him to do this or that, then with today's knowledge, one would call that "imperative voices" and judge it as a symptom of psychotic illness. Or if one reads in the Bible that Christ, hanging on the cross, had a lance rammed into his side by a Roman soldier and "blood and water" flowed out, then with today's knowledge one can assume that Christ must have had a haemorrhagic pleural effusion (a collection of blood and secretions between the lungs and ribs) at that time.

Thus, based on the descriptions in the Bible, one can surmise one disease or another. This does not mean that the assumptions I make in this book are necessarily correct. However, it seems more likely that many a miracle was a normal phenomenon and not due to supernatural influence by God.

Likewise, there are translation variants which seem more plausible than ones recognized by the Church as valid at present. For example, the description of the "virginity" of Mary, the Mother of God, is translated very differently. The Catholic Church assumes the "virgin birth" and translates the passage in Matthew "Behold, the virgin shall conceive a child, she shall bear a son..." (Mt 1:22) while non-theological interpreters assume that the translation should correctly read: "Behold, the young woman will conceive and bear a son..."[1] It is not intended to start a dispute here as to which translation or interpretation is the correct one, but it should serve as an example that even a slight change in translation can cause serious differences in the view and understanding of the Holy Scriptures and how supposed miracles can be "dissolved" by such small differences.

For me, the real miracle of Christian teaching is that even 2000 years ago Jesus preached views that we would still call very modern or revolutionary today. Renunciation of violence, love of neighbour, forgiveness, and the separation of church and state were unusual revolutionary thoughts at that time and represent the actual value of the Christian faith. Miracles may have served in the past to make the Christian doctrine "believable" to the less educated population. Christ was actually one of the first "modern" thinkers who also perceived marginalized persons as "human beings". Who wanted to see the idea of revenge replaced by charity. Who accepted the diversity of nature and saw it as a creation intended by God. All highly modern views. This is where the real miracle lies.

In the 21st century, however, it no longer seems appropriate to believe in supernatural miracles and to use them as "proof of truth" for a religion. We have learned in the course of history that many "facts" considered to be correct are quite wrong from today's point of view. While science has dealt with errors of interpretation that corresponded to the spirit of the times and corrected them over time, this is not the case with many religions. The reason often given for this rigidity of interpretation is the need for unchanging moral foundations. This may be partly true. However, we live in an age in which great problems await mankind and modern moral authorities would be in demand. Humans can interfere with creation by interfering with the genome and changing it forever. Artificial intelligence can take over human decisions, but is characterized by having no conscience. Medicine is not only replacing artificial limbs, but producing implants that interact with the brain, creating human-machine hybrids (cyborgs). The increasing exploitation of the world's resources and impending scarcity of resources increases the risk of unprecedented conflicts. While technical development is advancing rapidly, human moral and social development is lagging behind and unable to keep pace with new demands.

It is actually becoming more and more important that the churches or moral authorities stand up and establish and convey ethical and moral values adapted to the times, values that do justice to the problems of modern society and are not focused on problems that existed thousands of years ago. Problems of our time are not whether the pill may be taken or not, whether divorced people may go to communion or not, etc. Such thinking should actually come to an end in the third millennium. But this does not mean that religions should be abolished. No, there is a need for institutions that are independent of the state and that convey values and give comfort and a sense of life to people. The focus should not be on trivialities, not on temporary media hypes, but on the essentials that make us human beings and that do justice to the

[1] Translation error made Mary a virgin: Published 01/28/2009. https://www.welt.de/kultur/article3100214/Uebersetzungsfehler-machte-Maria-zur-Jungfrau.html.

common survival of mankind. And it must be finally recognized that there is no infallibility and no exclusivity claim to be the only salvific institution.

What is the purpose of this book? It is not about destroying Christians' faith. On the contrary. We have to realize that well-being can only be achieved by acting morally and ethically; that by doing so, we cause changes in our brain that ultimately benefit ourselves. Modern research shows us that God did not create man, but man created God (in his brain). In the human brain, there are predispositions to create a belief and that is good. We need faith to find our way in the world and to feel comfortable. But we do not need miracles. In the information age, we don't need religions that tell us fairy tales nor religious representatives who believe that one can prove God through so-called "miracles". The "holy" scriptures may have been helpful at a time when there were mainly oral traditions, when most people could neither write nor read. In the third millennium, however, ancient world views are outdated and moral precepts should be adapted to modern problems.

Of course, there is also the "danger" that many a dogma could be shaken. In the Middle Ages, these dogmas were defended with fire and sword. It must have been worth about 30 million human lives to the Roman Catholic Church to defend "its" doctrines—and the claims to power that went along with them. Wars, crusades, witch trials, the Inquisition, and incitement of the people against those of other faiths led to an extremely bloody church history.

In the late modern era, church doctrine is no longer defended with fire and flame, but with paper and pen. Instead of millions of dead people, there are now millions of people who are taken into psychological hostage. Bad conscience is an excellent means of manipulating people. In the long run, however, this strategy leads to mental illness and a sick society. Physical violence has turned into psychological violence in our society. But with this, the suffering of people has mutated from a "finite" misery to a "never-ending" misery. Divorced people, gays and lesbians, criminals or mentally ill people have no place anymore in many ecclesiastical societies (Christian Church). And yet, nature has provided for deviations from the norm, probably with a purpose.

As a physician who comes from a Catholic-influenced culture, I will refer only to the Bible in the following book. No attempt will be made to check the historical sources for their "correctness". That should be left to the historians. I will only try to "explain" single biblical texts from the point of view of a medical doctor. Thereby, as I said, I don't claim that the presented views are the only correct ones. Rather, they should stimulate discussion, discussions that are necessary to create a more contemporary reorganization, in order to give faith communities back the meaning they have had up to now and are increasingly losing in the modern age. Churches and faith communities would be more important than ever, especially in the present age, as guiding institutions for moral behaviour. However, the churches are no longer performing their actual tasks adequately. This is another reason why I have decided to cause a bit of trouble here with my interpretations, in the hope that by breaking up old thought structures, more space will be created again for modern, truly Christian thinking.

My special thanks go to my friends and discussion partners who contributed many ideas and helped me to write this book. In particular, I would like to thank J. G. Landers and Dorothy Butters, who provided a lot of constructive criticism and helped me with the translation into English.

Contents

Chapter 1
The Miracles in the New Testament

1.1 The Miracle of the Resurrection (The Execution of Jesus, Passion, Crucifixion and "Resurrection")

Some time between the year 30 and 36 AD, a man died whose death would change the world. Actually, it was not his death on the cross that caused such a stir, but the fact that he rose again from the dead three days after his execution. At least that's how the Bible tells it, and that's how about a billion people who call themselves Christians still believe it today. The very fact that someone could regain life by his own power after his execution represented something divine. In any case, the resurrection of Jesus Christ is one of the most important miracles in Christian doctrine. No other miracle is considered as important for believing Christians as the resurrection of Christ.

In contrast, there are some Non-Christians who believe that Christ did not really die on the cross, that he was only in suspended animation, and therefore could survive.[1] Yes, even resuscitation has been thought of, but this is very unlikely, since reanimation was not known until modern times and was certainly not practised in antiquity.

What really took place at the crucifixion site of Golgotha? At the place where Christ was crucified together with two other criminals? Is there any evidence in the Bible that could point to a survival of Jesus Christ? Clues that could explain the resurrection of Jesus Christ in a very simple way? The Gospel of John provides an amazingly accurate description of the passion of Jesus Christ. From his condemnation by Pontius Pilate, his torture by Roman soldiers, his journey to the execution site of

[1] Der Kreuzigungsbericht des Markusevangeliums Mk 15,20b–41. Johannes Schreiber, Walter de Gruyter-Verlag, Berlin 1986; books.google.at/books?hl=de&lr=&id=xZZsDwAAQBAJ&oi=fnd&pg=PR7&dq=Brandt+L+Scheintod+2016&ots=8NcFlZm9Bs&sig=9oGIRGVNvH02WaZRvGQ3PpfsKsQ#v=onepage&q&f=false.

M. Ledochowski, *The Miracles of the Bible Viewed Differently*,
https://doi.org/10.1007/978-3-031-51639-9_1

Golgotha, his crucifixion, and finally his burial. The descriptions are so exact that one can suspect one or the other damage to the tortured body on the basis of the described symptoms.

1.1.1 Blood Sweat, Jesus Sweats Blood

1.1.1.1 Original Text (Luke 22:39–46)

> **Jesus Prays on the Mount of Olives:** 39 And he came out and went, as was his custom, to the Mount of Olives, and the disciples followed him. 40 And when he came to the place, he said to them, "Pray that you may not enter into temptation." 41 And he withdrew from them about a stone's throw, and knelt down and prayed, 42 saying, "Father, if you are willing, remove this cup from me. Nevertheless, not my will, but yours, be done." 43 And there appeared to him an angel from heaven, strengthening him. 44 And being in agony he prayed more earnestly; and his sweat became like great drops of blood falling down to the ground. 45 And when he rose from prayer, he came to the disciples and found them sleeping for sorrow, 46 and he said to them, "Why are you sleeping? Rise and pray that you may not enter into temptation."

1.1.1.2 Description and Interpretation

Jesus had already allowed himself so many provocations that he was no longer acceptable to the high priests and the representatives of the Jewish religious community of that time. As a revolutionary preacher, Jesus was also a thorn in the side of the Roman occupying power. So it was easy for the Jewish elite, together with the Roman occupiers, to eliminate the hated itinerant preacher. They accused him and demanded his death. Jesus and his disciples were well aware of the approaching danger. So it came to the "last" supper, in which he said goodbye to his followers, so to speak. Afterwards, he still went with his disciples to the Mount of Olives for a final prayer, for Jesus was all too aware that he was about to be handed over to the Roman governor. Somewhat apart from his disciples, he gave free rein to his fear, praying to his God, seeing that his capture would only be a matter of time.

In this situation of enormous fear of death, sweat stood on his forehead. But not only that. The fear was so pronounced that he even had hallucinations and saw an angel. He prayed that he might be spared the foreseeable torments. But unfortunately without success, as the further story in the Bible tells us.

When he returned to his disciples, he saw with disappointment that they had fallen asleep. But the disciples noticed that the beads of sweat on his forehead were stained red. "Jesus was sweating blood" (Luke 22:44). This image has been put on canvas countless times by artists and represents well the human side of the Son of God. In the course of time, this image has even found its way into language when, in cases of extreme fear, one speaks of "someone sweating blood from fear."

The phenomenon of "sweating blood" actually exists. The medical profession calls it hematidrosis. Blood enters the sweat glands and is excreted with the sweat.[2] As a result, the sweat turns red and "blood drops" appear on the forehead, hands, feet, armpits and other areas with heavy sweating that are also well supplied with blood. Especially in people with autonomic lability, pronounced stress can lead to vasodilatation and an increase in vascular permeability. This can be so pronounced that even red blood cells can leak through the vessel wall and reach the surrounding tissue. If this affects the vessels of the sweat glands, these blood cells enter directly into the sweat glands and are excreted with the sweat.

But why does this not happen in every anxiety situation? Well, to a small extent it happens very often, because stress hormones such as adrenaline always lead to a widening of certain blood vessels and thus to an increased permeability of the vessel walls. This can be seen in the fact that many people experience swelling of the fingers or feet after physical exertion, during which adrenaline is also released. This swelling is also caused by dilated and more permeable vessels. In normal cases, however, the permeability is only so slight that only fluid leaks increasingly into the surrounding tissue. Only in very rare cases does the permeability of the vessels increase to such an extent that red blood cells can also escape. Sweating during stress is therefore normal. Sweating blood is already an indication of an excessive reaction of the body, an indication of an excessive reaction of the autonomic nervous system.

This phenomenon occurs again and again, as I said. One of the most famous cases from recent times was the world-famous Father Pius, who repeatedly exhibited stigmata during Mass celebrations: his palms turned red with blood-stained sweat. When he raised his arms to give his blessing to the church congregation, everyone could see it. He had the wound marks of Christ and was thus a "divine messenger". By a medical doctor, this would simply be called hematohidrosis in vegetative dystonia.

It can be assumed that many "saints", nuns or priests who received stigmata suffered from this phenomenon. The palms of the hands and soles of the feet are particularly densely covered with sweat glands, which is why hematohidrosis occurs most frequently here, followed later by the sweat glands on the forehead and face. Mental illnesses are usually accompanied by an enormous amount of stress, so that this phenomenon is more common in people with mental illnesses than in mentally healthy people.[3] On YouTube, you can watch movies about this rare but not unknown phenomenon.[4]

---

[2] Jerajani HR, Jaju B, Phiske MM, Lade N. Hematohidrosis—a rare clinical phenomenon. Indian J Dermatol. 2009 Jul;54(3):290-2. doi: https://doi.org/10.4103/0019-5154.55645. PMID: 20161867; PMCID: PMC2810702.

[3] Kluger N. Hematidrosis (bloody sweat): a review of the recent literature (1996–2016). Acta Dermatovenerol Alp Pannonica Adriat. 2018 Jun;27(2):85–90. PMID: 29945265.

[4] https://www.youtube.com/watch?v=FIug_C66DTw.

1.1.2 The Flagellation

1.1.2.1 Original Text (Mark 15:1; John 19:1)

Jesus Delivered to Pilate (Mark 15:1–15): 1 And as soon as it was morning, the chief priests held a consultation with the elders and scribes and the whole council. And they bound Jesus and led him away and delivered him over to Pilate. 2 And Pilate asked him, "Are you the King of the Jews?" And he answered him, "You have said so." 3 And the chief priests accused him of many things. 4 And Pilate again asked him, "Have you no answer to make? See how many charges they bring against you." 5 But Jesus made no further answer, so that Pilate was amazed.

Pilate Delivers Jesus to Be Crucified: 6 Now at the feast he used to release for them one prisoner for whom they asked. 7 And among the rebels in prison, who had committed murder in the insurrection, there was a man called Barabbas. 8 And the crowd came up and began to ask Pilate to do as he usually did for them. 9 And he answered them, saying, "Do you want me to release for you the King of the Jews?" 10 For he perceived that it was out of envy that the chief priests had delivered him up. 11 But the chief priests stirred up the crowd to have him release for them Barabbas instead. 12 And Pilate again said to them, "Then what shall I do with the man you call the King of the Jews?" 13 And they cried out again, "Crucify him." 14 And Pilate said to them, "Why? What evil has he done?" But they shouted all the more, "Crucify him." 15 So Pilate, wishing to satisfy the crowd, released for them Barabbas, and having scourged Jesus, he delivered him to be crucified.

Jesus Delivered to Be Crucified (John 19:1): 1 Then Pilate took Jesus and flogged him. 2 And the soldiers twisted together a crown of thorns and put it on his head and arrayed him in a purple robe. 3 They came up to him, saying, "Hail, King of the Jews!" and struck him with their hands. 4 Pilate went out again and said to them, "See, I am bringing him out to you that you may know that I find no guilt in him." 5 So Jesus came out, wearing the crown of thorns and the purple robe. Pilate said to them, "Behold the man!" 6 When the chief priests and the officers saw him, they cried out, "Crucify him, crucify him!" Pilate said to them, "Take him yourselves and crucify him, for I find no guilt in him." 7 The Jews answered him, "We have a law, and according to that law he ought to die because he has made himself the Son of God." 8 When Pilate heard this statement, he was even more afraid. 9 He entered his headquarters again and said to Jesus, "Where are you from?" But Jesus gave him no answer. 10 So Pilate said to him, "You will not speak to me? Do you not know that I have authority to release you and authority to crucify you?" 11 Jesus answered him, "You would have no authority over me at all unless it had been given you from above. Therefore, he who delivered me over to you has the greater sin." 12 From then on Pilate sought to release him, but the Jews cried out, "If you release this man, you are not Caesar's friend. Everyone who makes himself a king opposes Caesar." 13 So when Pilate heard these words, he brought Jesus out and sat down on the judgment seat at a place called The Stone Pavement, and in Aramaic Gabbatha. 14 Now it was the day of Preparation of the Passover. It was about the sixth hour. He said to the Jews, "Behold your King!" 15 They cried out, "Away with him, away with him, crucify him!" Pilate said to them, "Shall I crucify your King?" The chief priests answered, "We have no king but Caesar."

1.1.2.2 Description and Interpretation

Shortly after the episode of sweating blood, Christ was arrested on the Mount of Olives. By the famous "Judas kiss" he was betrayed by one of his disciples. Thus, the Roman soldiers knew whom to arrest. The next day, Jesus was accused before the Roman governor, Pontius Pilate. The latter was apparently not at all pleased about the accusation, but followed the pressure of the people and finally sentenced Jesus to death by crucifixion. To show that the sentence did not correspond to his inner conviction, he publicly washed his hands of it. Even today, the phrase "to wash one's hands in innocence" can be traced back to this incident described in the Bible.

Jesus was thus condemned and then taken away. He was thus at the mercy of the Roman soldiers. In the Bible, it is not only described how Jesus was mocked with a crown of thorns and by spitting on him, but also that he was scourged (see additional information). Often the prisoners met their death by this torture alone. In any case, this often resulted in massive injuries, especially to the rib cage, with broken ribs and internal bleeding.

Flagellation: The "flagrum", was an instrument of torture in the judicial system of the Roman Empire and was mainly used when the death penalty was imposed. Serious criminals were often scourged to death. In Christ's case, scourging (flagellation) was apparently used "only" as a torture. In scourging, unlike the whip, there were pieces of lead at the ends of the leather straps.

During flagellation, it was customary to tie the condemned to a stake in the ground and maltreat him with blows. It also happened that the condemned person died as a result of this flagellation.[5]

It can be assumed that during the scourging, one or another rib may have been broken. After all, humans are built in such a way that there were not only painful welts on the skin, but also injuries to the muscles and bones. When ribs break, this inevitably involves injury to the pleura and blood vessels. The injury to the blood vessels causes bleeding into the pleural cavity, which is the cavity between the ribs and the lungs. This results in what is known as a haemothorax,[6] an accumulation of blood between the ribs and lungs.

Another consequence of a pleural injury is the onset of an inflammatory response. Inflammatory reactions are actually part of a "healing repair" process that involves the formation of wound water (exudate). However, this healing process can lead to quite a few problems in this case, namely when the formation of wound water is so pronounced that it results in displacement of internal organs. When the formation of wound water is pronounced and accumulates in a cavity, the medical profession refers to it as an effusion or exudate. The exudate from a pleural injury can amount to several litres and usually flows into the pleural space, the cavity between the ribs and the lungs. This causes the lung on the affected side to become increasingly

[5] https://de.wikipedia.org/wiki/flagrum (Wikipedia 19.11.2021).

[6] Zeiler J, Idell S, Norwood S, Cook A. Hemothorax: A Review of the Literature. Clin Pulm Med. 2020 Jan;27(1):1–12. doi: https://doi.org/10.1097/CPM.0000000000000343. Epub 2020 Jan 10. PMID: 33437141; PMCID: PMC7799890.

compressed. Nowadays, we would call this a **pleural effusion**.[7] Both bleeding into the chest haemothorax and the inflammatory pleural effusion can progress to the point where the lungs are compressed to such an extent that the affected person can no longer breathe adequately. Especially in the case of bilateral effusions, the restriction of breathing can eventually even lead to death if timely therapy is not given. In any case, the affected person experiences shortness of breath. This is accompanied by an enormous drop in performance, because the lack of oxygen prevents the patient from performing sufficient muscle work, work that is above all necessary to maintain breathing.

The whole situation is made worse if there is constant bleeding further into the pleural cavity. This happens especially when the vessels of the thoracic wall have been injured, as was usually the case during flagellation. If a doctor were to puncture a pleural effusion in such a case, a "bloody, watery" fluid would appear. Such a mixture of wound water and bleeding is called a **haemorrhagic pleural effusion**. This type of pleural effusion is seen primarily after injury.[8] If it were just an inflammatory pleural effusion, the punctate would be a clear, sticky fluid. Therefore, when John's Gospel says that Jesus received a lance thrust in his side from a Roman soldier after his death and "blood and water" flowed out, we can assume that Jesus must have had a haemorrhagic pleural effusion at that time. However, this description says something else important: If blood and water flowed out, then the pleural effusion has obviously been successfully punctured! Thus, Jesus hanging on the cross has obviously unintentionally experienced a successful "therapy". The Roman soldier, of course, could not have known that he was performing a possibly life-saving relief puncture with his lance thrust. **The amazingly accurate description in the Bible shows us in a single sentence that there must have been a haemorrhagic pleural effusion and that a decompression puncture was performed**.

Today, trauma surgeons deal with pleural effusions primarily in the context of motor vehicle accidents. Injury-related pronounced *inflammatory* effusions are rarely seen today because the effusions usually cause such severe discomfort that the affected person goes immediately to the hospital for treatment.

In any case, a pleural effusion is not an uncommon phenomenon and is still seen by physicians today. The treatment of a pleural effusion, regardless of the cause, always consists of removing the pressure from the pleural space and performing a **decompression puncture**.[9] This is the prerequisite for the lungs to be able to expand again and for the affected person not to suffocate and to survive.

---

[7] Jany B, Welte T. Pleural Effusion in Adults-Etiology, Diagnosis, and Treatment. Dtsch Arztebl Int. 2019 May 24;116(21):377–386. doi: https://doi.org/10.3238/arztebl.2019.0377. PMID: 31315808; PMCID: PMC6647819.

[8] Capellier G, Gaussorgues P, Boyer F, Claud B, Robert D. [Diagnosis of post-traumatic pleural effusion]. Annales Francaises D'anesthesie et de Reanimation. 1989;8(2):131–132. DOI: https://doi.org/10.1016/s0750-7658(89)80165-0. PMID: 2735570.

[9] Ferreiro L, Porcel JM, Valdés L. Diagnosis and Management of Pleural Transudates. Arch Bronconeumol. 2017 Nov;53(11):629–636. English, Spanish. doi: https://doi.org/10.1016/j.arbres.2017.04.018. Epub 2017 Jun 19. PMID: 28641878.

1.1.3 The Way of the Cross

1.1.3.1 Original Text (Luke 23:26–42; Mark 15:21–32; Matthew 27:32–44)

The Crucifixion (Luke 23:26): 26 And as they led him away, they seized one Simon of Cyrene, who was coming in from the country, and laid on him the cross, to carry it behind Jesus. 27 And there followed him a great multitude of the people and of women, who were mourning and lamenting for him. 28 But turning to them, Jesus said, "Daughters of Jerusalem, do not weep for me, but weep for yourselves and for your children. 29 For behold, the days are coming when they will say, 'Blessed are the barren and the wombs that never bore and the breasts that never nursed!' 30 Then they will begin to say to the mountains, 'Fall on us,' and to the hills, 'Cover us.' 31 For if they do these things when the wood is green, what will happen when it is dry?" 32 Two others, who were criminals, were led away to be put to death with him. 33 And when they came to the place that is called The Skull, there they crucified him, and the criminals, one on his right and one on his left. 34 And Jesus said, "Father, forgive them, for they know not what they do." And they cast lots to divide his garments. 35 And the people stood by, watching, but the rulers scoffed at him, saying, "He saved others; let him save himself, if he is the Christ of God, his Chosen One!" 36 The soldiers also mocked him, coming up and offering him sour wine 37 and saying, "If you are the King of the Jews, save yourself!" 38 There was also an inscription over him, "This is the King of the Jews." 39 One of the criminals who were hanged railed at him, saying, "Are you not the Christ? Save yourself and us!" 40 But the other rebuked him, saying, "Do you not fear God, since you are under the same sentence of condemnation? 41 And we indeed justly, for we are receiving the due reward of our deeds; but this man has done nothing wrong." 42 And he said, "Jesus, remember me when you come into your kingdom." 43 And he said to him, "Truly, I say to you, today you will be with me in paradise."

The Crucifixion (Mark 15:21–32): 21 And they compelled a passer-by, Simon of Cyrene, who was coming in from the country, the father of Alexander and Rufus, to carry his cross. 22 And they brought him to the place called Golgotha (which means Place of a Skull). 23 And they offered him wine mixed with myrrh, but he did not take it. 24 And they crucified him and divided his garments among them, casting lots for them, to decide what each should take. 25 And it was the third hour when they crucified him. 26 And the inscription of the charge against him read, "The King of the Jews." 27 And with him, they crucified two robbers, one on his right and one on his left. 29 And those who passed by derided him, wagging their heads and saying, "Aha! You who would destroy the temple and rebuild it in three days, 30 save yourself, and come down from the cross!" 31 So also the chief priests with the scribes mocked him to one another, saying, "He saved others; he cannot save himself. 32 Let the Christ, the King of Israel, come down now from the cross that we may see and believe." Those who were crucified with him also reviled him.

The Crucifixion (Matthew 27:32–44): 32 As they went out, they found a man of Cyrene, Simon by name. They compelled this man to carry his cross. 33 And when they came to a place called Golgotha (which means Place of a Skull), 34 they offered him wine to drink, mixed with gall, but when he tasted it, he would not drink it. 35 And when they had crucified him, they divided his garments among them by casting lots. 36 Then they sat down and kept watch over him there. 37 And over his head they put the charge against him, which read, "This is Jesus, the King of the Jews." 38 Then two robbers were crucified with him, one on the right and one on the left. 39 And those who passed by derided him, wagging their heads 40 and saying, "You who would destroy the temple and rebuild it in three days, save yourself! If you are the Son of God, come down from the cross." 41 So also the chief priests, with the scribes and elders, mocked him, saying, 42 "He saved others; he cannot save himself. He is the King of Israel; let him come down now from the cross, and we will believe in him. 43 He trusts in God; let God deliver him now, if he desires him. For he said, 'I am the Son of God.'" 44 And the robbers who were crucified with him also reviled him in the same way.

1.1.3.2 Description and Interpretation

The crucifixion took place just outside Jerusalem, at a place called Golgotha. The prisoners had to carry their crosses there themselves. This was done with the participation of an excited population, most of whom must have enjoyed it. In any case, one can well imagine the spectacle of such a "crusade" and the imminent execution.

Just like the other two condemned men, Christ had to load up his cross and carry it all the way to Golgotha. In the process, an unforeseen event occurred, for the Bible states that Christ's cross was eventually loaded onto a stranger. Apparently, the Via Dolorosa stalled because Jesus was no longer able to carry his cross. So Jesus' cross was simply loaded onto another man standing by the roadside. The stranger who was coerced into carrying Jesus' cross is even known by name. His name was Simon of Cyrene, and he entered history through this incident. In any case, it can be assumed that the Roman soldiers were not concerned with sparing the prisoner, but with ensuring that there was no further delay in the execution of the sentence.

From a medical point of view, it is important to note that Jesus did not manage to carry his cross himself, while the other condemned men apparently did.

This is another sign that **Jesus' oxygen supply was already poor**, so that even under threat of pain, **he was no longer able to provide the muscular effort necessary to carry his cross**. The other prisoners, who may have suffered lesser thoracic injuries as they may have not been flagellated so hard, were able to cope. They were able to carry their crosses up the mountain without any problem. This is a sign that the pleural effusion must have been quite advanced in Christ on his "way of the cross". In any case, it is well described in the Bible that Jesus Christ, in spite of effort, could not perform as well as the other condemned prisoners. Thus, it is clear from the Bible text that **Jesus' cardio-respiratory performance was already limited on the way to Golgotha**.

The Way of the Cross ("Via Dolorosa"), as described by the Catholic Church, contains 14 stations. Stations 3 through 5 depict the Way of the Cross as follows (the teaching of the Roman Catholic Church differs significantly from the Bible here):

Station 3: **Jesus falls for the first time under the cross (not mentioned in the Bible)**: The soldiers drive Jesus through the streets of Jerusalem, and under the weight of the heavy wooden cross he collapses. But the soldiers force him to go on.

4th station: **Jesus meets his mother (not mentioned in the Bible)**: Among the many people standing on the roadside watching Jesus Christ carry the cross to the place of execution in great pain is his mother Mary. The closeness and love of his mother gives Jesus the strength and courage to continue on the difficult path.

5th station: **Simon of Cyrene helps Jesus to carry the cross (mentioned in the Bible: Mt. 27,32)**: Jesus is getting weaker and weaker and can hardly carry it. So the soldiers order the farmer Simon of Cyrene to carry the cross.

6th station: **Veronica hands Jesus the face-cloth (not mentioned in the Bible)**: According to this, St. Veronica handed her cloth to Jesus Christ on his way to Golgotha to wipe the sweat and blood from his face. In the process, Jesus' face is said to have miraculously imprinted itself on the sweat cloth as a so-called Veronica image.

1.1.4 The Crucifixion and Death of Jesus

1.1.4.1 Original Text (Luke 23:33–49; Mark 15:21–41; Matthew 27:45–56; John 19:16–37)

The Crucifixion (Luke 23:33–49): 26 And as they led him away, they seized one Simon of Cyrene, who was coming in from the country, and laid on him the cross, to carry it behind Jesus. 27 And there followed him a great multitude of the people and of women, who were mourning and lamenting for him. 28 But turning to them, Jesus said, "Daughters of Jerusalem, do not weep for me, but weep for yourselves and for your children. 29 For behold, the days are coming when they will say, 'Blessed are the barren and the wombs that never bore and the breasts that never nursed!' 30 Then they will begin to say to the mountains, 'Fall on us,' and to the hills, 'Cover us.' 31 For if they do these things when the wood is green, what will happen when it is dry?" 32 Two others, who were criminals, were led away to be put to death with him. 33 And when they came to the place that is called The Skull, there they crucified him, and the criminals, one on his right and one on his left. 34 And Jesus said, "Father, forgive them, for they know not what they do." And they cast lots to divide his garments. 35 And the people stood by, watching, but the rulers scoffed at him, saying, "He saved others; let him save himself, if he is the Christ of God, his Chosen One!" 36 The soldiers also mocked him, coming up and offering him sour wine 37 and saying, "If you are the King of the Jews, save yourself!" 38 There was also an inscription over him, "This is the King of the Jews." 39 One of the criminals who were hanged railed at him, saying, "Are you not the Christ? Save yourself and us!" 40 But the other rebuked him, saying, "Do you not fear God, since you are under the same sentence of condemnation? 41 And we indeed justly, for we are receiving the due reward of our deeds; but this man has done nothing wrong." 42 And he said, "Jesus, remember me when you come into your kingdom." 43 And he said to him, "Truly, I say to you, today you will be with me in paradise." **The Death of Jesus:** 44 It was now about the sixth hour, and there was darkness over the whole land until the ninth hour, 45 while the sun's light failed. And the curtain of the temple was torn in two. 46 Then Jesus, calling out with a loud voice, said, "Father, into your hands I commit my spirit!" And having said this, he breathed his last. 47 Now when the centurion saw what had taken place, he praised God, saying, "Certainly this man was innocent!" 48 And all the crowds that had assembled for this spectacle, when they saw what had taken place, returned home beating their breasts. 49 And all his acquaintances and the women who had followed him from Galilee stood at a distance watching these things.

The Crucifixion (Mark 15:21–41): 21 And they compelled a passer-by, Simon of Cyrene, who was coming in from the country, the father of Alexander and Rufus, to carry his cross. 22 And they brought him to the place called Golgotha (which means Place of a Skull). 23 And they offered him wine mixed with myrrh, but he did not take it. 24 And they crucified him and divided his garments among them, casting lots for them, to decide what each should take. 25 And it was the third hour when they crucified him. 26 And the inscription of the charge against him read, "The King of the Jews." 27 And with him, they crucified two robbers, one on his right and one on his left. 29 And those who passed by derided him, wagging their heads and saying, "Aha! You who would destroy the temple and rebuild it in three days, 30 save yourself, and come down from the cross!" 31 So also the chief priests with the scribes mocked him to one another, saying, "He saved others; he cannot save himself. 32 Let the Christ, the King of Israel, come down now from the cross that we may see and believe." Those who were crucified with him also reviled him. **The Death of Jesus:** 33 And when the sixth hour had come, there was darkness over the whole land until the ninth hour. 34 And at the ninth hour Jesus cried with a loud voice, "Eloi, Eloi, lema sabachtani?" which means, "My God, my God, why have you forsaken me?" 35 And some of the bystanders hearing it said, "Behold, he is calling Elijah." 36 And someone ran and filled a sponge with sour wine, put it on a reed and gave it to him to drink, saying, "Wait, let us see whether Elijah will come to take him down." 37 And Jesus uttered a loud cry and breathed his last. 38 And the curtain of the temple was torn in two, from top to bottom. 39 And when the centurion, who stood facing him, saw that in this way he breathed his last, he said, "Truly this man was the Son[9] of God!" 40 There were also women looking on from a distance, among whom were Mary Magdalene, and Mary the mother of James the younger and of Joses, and Salome. 41 When he was in Galilee, they followed him and ministered to him, and there were also many other women who came up with him to Jerusalem.

The Crucifixion (Matthew 27:45–56): 32 As they went out, they found a man of Cyrene, Simon by name. They compelled this man to carry his cross. 33 And when they came to a place called Golgotha (which means Place of a Skull), 34 they offered him wine to drink, mixed with gall, but when he tasted it, he would not drink it. 35 And when they had crucified him, they divided his garments among them by casting lots. 36 Then they sat down and kept watch over him there. 37 And over his head they put the charge against him, which read, "This is Jesus, the King of the Jews." 38 Then two robbers were crucified with him, one on the right and one on the left. 39 And those who passed by derided him, wagging their heads 40 and saying, "You who would destroy the temple and rebuild it in three days, save yourself! If you are the Son of God, come down from the cross." 41 So also the chief priests, with the scribes and elders, mocked him, saying, 42 "He saved others; he cannot save himself. He is the King of Israel; let him come down now from the cross, and we will believe in him. 43 He trusts in God; let God deliver him now, if he desires him. For he said, 'I am the Son of God.'" 44 And the robbers who were crucified with him also reviled him in the same way. **The Death of Jesus:** 45 Now from the sixth hour there was darkness over all the land until the ninth hour. 46 And about the ninth hour, Jesus cried out with a loud voice, saying, "Eli, Eli, lema sabachtani?" that is, "My God, my God, why have you forsaken me?" 47 And some of the bystanders, hearing it, said, "This man is calling Elijah." 48 And one of them at once ran and took a sponge, filled it with sour wine, and put it on a reed and gave it to him to drink. 49 But the others said, "Wait, let us see whether Elijah will come to save him." 50 And Jesus cried out again with a loud voice and yielded up his spirit. 51 And behold, the curtain of the temple was torn in two, from top to bottom. And the earth shook, and the rocks were split. 52 The tombs also were opened. And many bodies of the saints who had fallen asleep were raised, 53 and coming out of the tombs after his resurrection, they went into the holy city and appeared to many. 54 When the centurion and those who were with him, keeping watch over Jesus, saw the earthquake and what took place, they were filled with awe and said, "Truly this was the Son of God!" 55 There were also many women there, looking on from a distance, who had followed Jesus from Galilee, ministering to him, 56 among whom were Mary Magdalene and Mary the mother of James and Joseph and the mother of the sons of Zebedee.

The Crucifixion (John 19:16–37): 16 So he delivered him over to them to be crucified. So they took Jesus, 17 and he went out, bearing his own cross, to the place called The Place of a Skull, which in Aramaic is called Golgotha. 18 There they crucified him, and with him two others, one on either side, and Jesus between them. 19 Pilate also wrote an inscription and put it on the cross. It read, "Jesus of Nazareth, the King of the Jews." 20 Many of the Jews read this inscription, for the place where Jesus was crucified was near the city, and it was written in Aramaic, in Latin, and in Greek. 21 So the chief priests of the Jews said to Pilate, "Do not write, 'The King of the Jews,' but rather, 'This man said, I am King of the Jews.'" 22 Pilate answered, "What I have written, I have written." 23 When the soldiers had crucified Jesus, they took his garments and divided them into four parts, one part for each soldier; also his tunic. But the tunic was seamless, woven in one piece from top to bottom, 24 so they said to one another, "Let us not tear it, but cast lots for it to see whose it shall be." This was to fulfill the Scripture which says, "They divided my garments among them, and for my clothing they cast lots." So the soldiers did these things, 25 but standing by the cross of Jesus were his mother and his mother's sister, Mary the wife of Clopas, and Mary Magdalene. 26 When Jesus saw his mother and the disciple whom he loved standing nearby, he said to his mother, "Woman, behold, your son!" 27 Then he said to the disciple, "Behold, your mother!" And from that hour, the disciple took her to his own home. **The Death of Jesus:** 28 After this, Jesus, knowing that all was now finished, said (to fulfill the Scripture), "I thirst." 29 A jar full of sour wine stood there, so they put a sponge full of the sour wine on a hyssop branch and held it to his mouth. 30 When Jesus had received the sour wine, he said, "It is finished," and he bowed his head and gave up his spirit. **Jesus' Side Is Pierced:** 31 Since it was the day of Preparation, and so that the bodies would not remain on the cross on the Sabbath (for that Sabbath was a high day), the Jews asked Pilate that their legs might be broken and that they might be taken away. 32 So the soldiers came and broke the legs of the first, and of the other who had been crucified with him. 33 But when they came to Jesus and saw that he was already dead, they did not break his legs. 34 But one of the soldiers pierced his side with a spear, and at once there came out blood and water. 35 He who saw it has borne witness—his testimony is true, and he knows that he is telling the truth—that you also may believe. 36 For these things took place that the Scripture might be fulfilled: "Not one of his bones will be broken." 37 And again another Scripture says, "They will look on him whom they have pierced."

1.1.4.2 Description and Interpretation

Jesus carried his cross, or rather had Simon of Cyrene carry it, to Mount Golgotha. Once there, Christ was nailed to the cross before it was erected. With the erection of the cross, the circulatory situation inevitably worsened. Hanging on the cross, oxygen required for breathing work is increased, one gets little air and breathes heavily. In crucifixion, death actually occurs by "suffocation", because the oxygen required by the respiratory muscles is greater than one can absorb in the same time by breathing. Thus, with each breath, there is a small increase in the lack of oxygen. It's a cruel death, because suffocation occurs very slowly, and it can take days to die. If one is lucky, so much blood pools in the legs that it causes circulatory problems to the brain and one becomes unconscious. With this, one still lives on, but one no longer suffers because consciousness is eliminated.

This imbalance of respiratory work to oxygen intake can be made even worse by breaking the legs of the crucified person, because this finally eliminates the ability to push the body upwards, with his feet that were nailed to the cross, relieving the strain on the auxiliary respiratory muscles and the crucified person must finally die. If the dying process took too long or was too slow for the Roman soldiers, then the legs of those hanging on the cross were broken because experience showed that the onset of death can be significantly accelerated by breaking the legs. In the case of Jesus Christ, however, the legs were NOT broken (John 19:33), an essential condition for Jesus to remain alive.

It is reasonable to assume that bloody exudate continued to pour into the pleural cavity during the course of the crucifixion. Such a **redistribution of fluid from the blood vessels into the so-called transcellular space** (see additional information) leads to severe thirst. The thirst occurs primarily because fluid is "lost" from the circulation by running into the pleural space. This changes the osmotic pressure in the blood, which in turn **causes excruciating thirst**. This symptom is also described in the Gospel: "I thirst. A vessel full of vinegar was standing there. They put a sponge full of vinegar on a hyssop branch and held it to his mouth (John 19:28–29)." The vinegar offered, however, did not really make up for the loss of fluids.

As the pleural effusion progresses, there is not only a decrease in oxygen saturation in the blood, but more importantly a rise in CO_2 (**hypercapnia**).[10] A rise in CO_2 occurs because carbon dioxide can no longer be adequately exhaled. In such a case, unconsciousness is caused less by the drop in oxygen than by the rise in CO_2 (**so-called CO_2 narcosis**). If breathing is disturbed, e.g., by a pleural effusion, hypercapnia initially causes an increased respiratory drive: the body tries to breathe off the excess CO_2 by increased respiratory effort, and one subjectively develops the feeling of respiratory distress. Having reached this point, Jesus cries out once again with the last of his strength, as the Bible states "But Jesus cried out once more with a loud voice. Then he breathed out the Spirit! (Matthew 27:50)." With this, Jesus has used up his last reserve of breath. As a result, he is no longer able to breathe out the accumulated CO_2 sufficiently, so that he becomes unconscious.

Unconsciousness is not only the result of oxygen deficiency but mainly a result of CO_2 narcosis[11]: It is important to note here that although unconsciousness occurs during CO_2 narcosis, the oxygen tension is still easily sufficient to maintain

[10] Kreppein U, Litterst P, Westhoff M. Hyperkapnisches Atemversagen. Pathophysiologie, Beatmungsindikationen und -durchführung [Hypercapnic respiratory failure. Pathophysiology, indications for mechanical ventilation and management]. Med Klin Intensivmed Notfmed. 2016 Apr;111(3):196–201. German. doi: https://doi.org/10.1007/s00063-016-0143-2. Epub 2016 Feb 22. PMID: 26902369.

[11] Duan J, Han X, Bai L, Zhou L, Huang S. Assessment of heart rate, acidosis, consciousness, oxygenation, and respiratory rate to predict noninvasive ventilation failure in hypoxemic patients. Intensive Care Med. 2017 Feb;43(2):192–199. doi: https://doi.org/10.1007/s00134-016-4601-3. Epub 2016 Nov 3. PMID: 27812731.

the function of vital organs.[12] With prolonged CO_2-narcosis, respiratory paralysis and the onset of death by suffocation would eventually occur. **This transition from unconsciousness without respiratory arrest and unconsciousness with respiratory arrest and the associated asphyxiation to the onset of death is not easy to recognize even for a modern physician.** It may therefore be doubted that it was possible for the Roman soldiers and the assembled people over 2000 years ago to notice this difference.

Since there have been repeated misinterpretations of death, there are now guidelines for physicians for the safe determination of death.[13] Definite signs of death occur at the earliest 1 h after death, but usually not until 6 h after death. These include, most notably, rigor mortis and death-marks. In the case of Christ, this time period was apparently never reached on the cross. His body was removed from the cross relatively soon after the crucifixion, or after his "death," and placed in the tomb (Matthew 27:57–59). This period of time, however, was not sufficient to establish certain death. This might also have been the reason the Roman soldier, who had to keep guard in front of the cross, stabbed Jesus, who was hanging on the cross, in the side with his lance. It served to "make sure" that Christ was dead for sure and could not survive. In the Gospel of John, this process is described as follows: "But one of the soldiers pierced his side with a spear, and at once there came out blood and water." (John 19:34). The presence of a haemorrhagic pleural effusion cannot be described more beautifully. If after a stab in the side, "blood and water flowed out," then there MUST have been a pleural effusion. However, the treatment of a pleural effusion—even today—is to puncture the effusion. This is exactly what the Roman soldier did unintentionally with his lance thrust. It can therefore be assumed that the soldier's lance thrust was accidentally a life-saving measure, and that Jesus was able to survive as a result.

Nowadays, when patients are admitted comatose in such a condition treated by a decompression puncture, they usually do not regain consciousness immediately. It often takes several hours until the CO_2 dissolved in the brain is redistributed, and the brain has recovered in such a way that the patient "wakes up" again.[14] A similar process is likely to have occurred with Christ. In addition, cerebral oedema may have developed in the context of oxygen deprivation and hypercapnia, which was slow to resolve and therefore delayed regaining consciousness after successful "treatment".[15]

---

[12] Benghanem S, Mazeraud A, Azabou E, Chhor V, Shinotsuka CR, Claassen J, Rohaut B, Sharshar T. Brainstem dysfunction in critically ill patients. Crit Care. 2020 Jan 6;24(1):5. doi: https://doi.org/10.1186/s13054-019-2718-9. PMID: 31907011; PMCID: PMC6945639.

[13] Weckbecker, K., Bleckwenn, M. Leichenschau und Todesbescheinigung durch den Hausarzt: Probleme beim Bescheinigen vor Ort. Bundesgesundheitsbl 62, 1446–1451 (2019). https://doi.org/10.1007/s00103-019-03044-3.

[14] Joyce RR, McGee WT. Hypercapnic cerebral edema presenting in a woman with asthma: a case report. J Med Case Rep. 2011 May 20;5:192. doi: https://doi.org/10.1186/1752-1947-5-192. PMID: 21599887; PMCID: PMC3113998.

[15] Roh D, Merkler AE, Al-Mufti F, Morris N, Agarwal S, Claassen J, Park S. Global cerebral edema from hypercapnic respiratory acidosis and response to hyperosmolar therapy. Neurology.

The transcellular space is the fluid space located outside the blood vessels and the intercellular space in the body cavities lined with epithelia. It is a part of the extracellular space. The transcellular space includes body cavities such as:

- Pleura
- Peritoneum
- Pericardium (heart sac)
- CSF spaces (brain)
- Cavities such as lumina of the
  - gastrointestinal tract,
  - urogenital system, and the
  - glands.

1.1.5 The Burial of the Body

1.1.5.1 Original Text (Matthew 27:57–61; John 19:38–42; Mark 15:42–47)

Jesus Is Buried (Matthew 27:57–61): 57 When it was evening, there came a rich man from Arimathea, named Joseph, who also was a disciple of Jesus. 58 He went to Pilate and asked for the body of Jesus. Then Pilate ordered it to be given to him. 59 And Joseph took the body and wrapped it in a clean linen shroud 60 and laid it in his own new tomb, which he had cut in the rock. And he rolled a great stone to the entrance of the tomb and went away. 61 Mary Magdalene and the other Mary were there, sitting opposite the tomb.

Jesus Is Buried (John 19:38–42): 38 After these things Joseph of Arimathea, who was a disciple of Jesus, but secretly for fear of the Jews, asked Pilate that he might take away the body of Jesus, and Pilate gave him permission. So he came and took away his body. 39 Nicodemus also, who earlier had come to Jesus by night, came bringing a mixture of myrrh and aloes, about seventy-five pounds in weight. 40 So they took the body of Jesus and bound it in linen cloths with the spices, as is the burial custom of the Jews. 41 Now in the place where he was crucified there was a garden, and in the garden a new tomb in which no one had yet been laid. 42 So because of the Jewish day of Preparation, since the tomb was close at hand, they laid Jesus there.

Jesus Is Buried (Mark 15:42–47): 42 And when evening had come, since it was the day of Preparation, that is, the day before the Sabbath, 43 Joseph of Arimathea, a respected member of the council, who was also himself looking for the kingdom of God, took courage and went to Pilate and asked for the body of Jesus. 44 Pilate was surprised to hear that he should have already died. And summoning the centurion, he asked him whether he was already dead. 45

2016 Apr 19;86(16):1556–8. doi: https://doi.org/10.1212/WNL.0000000000002584. Epub 2016 Mar 18. PMID: 26992857; PMCID: PMC4836882.

And when he learned from the centurion that he was dead, he granted the corpse to Joseph. 46 And Joseph bought a linen shroud, and taking him down, wrapped him in the linen shroud and laid him in a tomb that had been cut out of the rock. And he rolled a stone against the entrance of the tomb. 47 Mary Magdalene and Mary the mother of Joses saw where he was laid.

1.1.5.2 Description and Interpretation

Jesus was hanging unconscious on the cross. Since his legs were not broken, a soldier pierced his side with his lance, and plenty of fluid flowed out of his body. This allowed the lungs to expand somewhat and the respiratory situation improved hour by hour.

After a decompression puncture, there is initially a better supply of oxygen. Although CO_2 is also exhaled more at the same time, it still takes time before consciousness is regained. This delayed awakening is due to the fact that the carbon dioxide present in the brain often takes several hours to be excreted. Time enough for the relatives to go to the governor and request the early removal of the body from the cross (Matthew 27:57–61). Since the next day was the Sabbath, a holy day on which the Jews were not allowed to work, this was another reason for approval by the governor. Christ was "dead." The people had had their spectacle and an example had been made by the Roman side, so there was no longer any reason not to comply with the wishes of the relatives. Thus, the body was removed from the cross prematurely and Christ was placed in what was presumably a cool tomb.

Whether it was really the Sabbath that caused the relatives to make such haste to obtain the release of the body, or whether the relatives perhaps realized that Christ may not have been quite dead yet, is an open question. What is certain is that Christ was taken down from the cross in a TIMELY manner, that is, relatively soon after his "death" (Matthew 27:57–60), thus making another exception to the usual process of crucifixion. This further enhanced his chances of survival.

The Bible even states the exact manner in which the "corpse" was further cared for. Even quantities were not omitted: "Nicodemus also came, who had once visited Jesus by night. He brought a mixture of myrrh and aloes, about a hundred pounds. They took the body of Jesus and wrapped it with linen bandages, together with the fragrant ointments, as is the custom at the Jewish burial" (John 19:39–40).

Substances were used which exerted strong pharmacological effects on the vessels, haemostasis, and inflammation. Just what a battered but still living body needed. Also, the coolness of the tomb and the wrapping in linen bandages, which contributed to the compression of the vessels and thus may have had a circulatory stabilizing effect, represented favourable circumstances to accelerate the recovery process. **In any case, a survival of Jesus Christ seems quite possible and even probable under the given conditions**. The respective steps that allow this assumption are described in the Bible with astonishing accuracy.

Abstract: Diagnoses: From today's point of view, it must be assumed that Jesus Christ suffered injuries to the ribs (ICD[16]-10: S22.3) and subsequently a traumatic haemorrhagic pleural effusion (ICD-10: J90) as a result of the scourging. As a result, respiratory failure (ICD-10: J96.0) with CO2 narcosis (ICD-10: J96.91) and presumed death occurred. Due to Longinus' lance puncture, he was unknowingly given a decompression puncture and thus "properly treated". Jesus thus underwent a life-saving therapeutic intervention (ICD-10: 8–152.1).

- Effects of aloe and myrrh (Doccheck retrieved 26/07/2019):
  - Astringent (contracting vessels and thus stabilizing circulation),
  - anti-inflammatory,
  - analgesic, disinfecting and
  - haemostatic
- Effects of Aloe:
  - anti-inflammatory,
  - antiphlogistic,
  - among others.

1.2 The Birth of John the Baptist, Foretold (The Story of Zechariah)

1.2.1 Original Text (Luke 1:5–25)

Birth of John the Baptist Foretold (Luke 1:5–25): 5 In the days of Herod, king of Judea, there was a priest named Zechariah, of the division of Abijah. And he had a wife from the daughters of Aaron, and her name was Elizabeth. 6 And they were both righteous before God, walking blamelessly in all the commandments and statutes of the Lord. 7 But they had no child, because Elizabeth was barren, and both were advanced in years. 8 Now while he was serving as priest before God when his division was on duty, 9 according to the custom of the priesthood, he was chosen by lot to enter the temple of the Lord and burn incense. 10 And the whole multitude of the people were praying outside at the hour of incense. 11 And there appeared to him an angel of the Lord standing on the right side of the altar of incense. 12 And Zechariah was troubled when he saw him, and fear fell upon him. 13 But the angel said to him, "Do not be afraid, Zechariah, for your prayer has been heard, and your wife Elizabeth will bear you a son, and you shall call his name John. 14 And you will have joy and gladness, and many will rejoice at his birth, 15 for he will be great before the Lord. And he must not drink wine or strong drink, and he will be filled with the Holy Spirit, even from his mother's womb. 16 And he will turn many of the children of Israel to the Lord their God, 17 and he will go before him in the spirit and power of Elijah, to turn the hearts of the fathers to the children, and the disobedient to the wisdom of the just, to make ready for the Lord a

[16] ICD: International Classification of Diseases.

people prepared." 18 And Zechariah said to the angel, "How shall I know this? For I am an old man, and my wife is advanced in years." 19 And the angel answered him, "I am Gabriel. I stand in the presence of God, and I was sent to speak to you and to bring you this good news. 20 And behold, you will be silent and unable to speak until the day that these things take place, because you did not believe my words, which will be fulfilled in their time." 21 And the people were waiting for Zechariah, and they were wondering at his delay in the temple. 22 And when he came out, he was unable to speak to them, and they realized that he had seen a vision in the temple. And he kept making signs to them and remained mute. 23 And when his time of service was ended, he went to his home. 24 After these days his wife Elizabeth conceived, and for five months she kept herself hidden, saying, 25 "Thus the Lord has done for me in the days when he looked on me, to take away my reproach among people."

1.2.2 Description and Interpretation

The story of Zechariah is told in the Gospel of Luke and takes place shortly before the birth of Christ. A Jewish priest, he was married to Elizabeth of the house of Aaron. The Bible tells us that he was childless, which apparently worried him quite a bit, especially since he and his wife Elizabeth were already advanced in age. One day he was assigned to temple duty for the annual feast to offer the **incense sacrifice**. This was an honourable task. While he was offering the incense and the faithful were waiting, **he saw an angel on the right side of the altar. The angel began to speak** and told him that despite his old age, he could still become a father and have the son he so longed for. The angel said: "Do not be afraid, Zechariah, for your supplication has been heard, and your wife Elizabeth will bear you a son, and you shall call his name John". **Zechariah was obviously not so sure about the apparition** and wanted to know from the angel who he was and also demanded a sure sign that the whole apparition was not a mirage, but a real experience. The angel introduced himself as Archangel Gabriel. As a sign that the experience had actually taken place and was not a mirage, he **afflicted Zechariah with muteness**. Apparently, the dialogue between Zechariah and the angel lasted quite a long time, because the people waiting in front of the temple became quite impatient. The Bible also gives details of the conversation between Zechariah and the angel Gabriel. When Zechariah stepped in front of the temple to give his blessing to the believers, he realized that he could no longer speak. So he simply waved to the faithful and went home. The muteness continued until the birth of his son John (the Baptist), or the day of his circumcision.

When someone sees apparitions, that is, sees something that is not objectively there, we speak of **visual hallucinations**.[17] If one additionally hears voices that are objectively not there, one speaks of **auditory hallucinations**.[18]

[17] Coerver KA, Subramanian PS. Visual hallucinations in psychiatric, neurologic, and ophthalmologic disease. Curr Opin Ophthalmol. 2020 Nov;31(6):475-482. doi: https://doi.org/10.1097/ICU.0000000000000701. PMID: 33009079.

[18] Blom JD. Auditory hallucinations. Handb Clin Neurol. 2015;129:433–55. doi: https://doi.org/10.1016/B978-0-444-62630-1.00024-X. PMID: 25726283.

If the hallucinatory experiences become so pronounced that one can even converse with these apparitions and a dialogue takes place, this is called "dialogizing voices". Dialogizing voices are among the first-order symptoms, and visual as well as auditory hallucinations are among the second-order symptoms for the diagnosis of schizophrenia.[19] By themselves, they would meet the criteria for a diagnosis of schizophrenia and, according to the DSM-5, allow a diagnosis of schizophrenia.[20] That the content of dialogizing voices is mainly about topics that are also otherwise "on the mind" of the affected person is a common observation. It is therefore understandable that the "conversation between Zechariah and the angel Gabriel" was about the unsolved problem of Zechariah's lack of offspring, since time was pressing because he and his wife were already of advanced age. Also, the "**inability to speak**", is a not so rare accompanying phenomenon of many psychiatric illnesses and can occur especially after an acute schizophrenic episode[21] and persist as "schizophrenic residual" (F20.5) for prolonged periods of time, even months. In medicine, this phenomenon is called **mutism**[22] and is defined as "psychologically induced silence of a person, without defect of the speech organ or organs." Speech and **speechlessness has a lot to do with the psyche and psychological stress situations**. This can be seen from figures of speech: When someone is exposed to high stress, and maybe they get shocked, very sad or quite unbelievable information they are suddenly "speechless" or "can't find words" or "it makes them speechless". How often do you hear on TV after an attack with many dead people the words of the commentators or politicians "I am at a loss for words". In any case, short-term speechlessness is a well-known phenomenon and probably occurs more frequently in people with a tendency to depression or schizophrenia than in manic people who are "quick-witted" and always have an immediate answer ready.

But how did this instance of a schizophrenic episode come about? The Bible offers an answer to this as well: Luke describes that Zechariah offered a **smoking sacrifice**. In the case of smoke offerings, incense and other fragrant substances were added at that time and are still added today, which can also have hallucinogenic effects in high concentrations.[23] Incentol, which comes from incense, has a strong hallucinogenic effect and is similar to LSD, which is better known today. How the

---

[19] Tandon, Rajiv, et al. "Definition and description of schizophrenia in the DSM-5." Schizophr. Res., vol. 150, no. 1, Oct. 2013, pp. 3–10. doi: https://doi.org/10.1016/j.schres.2013.05.028.

[20] American Psychiatric Association's (2013) *Diagnostic and Statistical Manual of Mental Disorders* (5th ed.; DSM-5).

[21] Vani, Pulaparambil, et al. "Mutism as a component of obsessive-compulsive symptoms in patients with schizophrenia: A report of two cases." Asian J. Psychiatr., vol. 54, Dec. 2020, p. 102337.. doi: https://doi.org/10.1016/j.ajp.2020.102337.

[22] Rozenek EB, Orlof W, Nowicka ZM, Wilczyńska K, Waszkiewicz N. Selective mutism - an overview of the condition and etiology: is the absence of speech just the tip of the iceberg? Psychiatr Pol. 2020 Apr 30;54(2):333–349. English, Polish. doi: https://doi.org/10.12740/PP/OnlineFirst/108503. Epub 2020 Apr 30. PMID: 32772064.

[23] Dannaway FR. Strange fires, weird smokes and psychoactive combustibles: entheogens and incense in ancient traditions. J Psychoactive Drugs. 2010 Dec;42(4):485–97. doi: https://doi.org/10.1080/02791072.2010.10400711. PMID: 21305913.

hallucinogenic effect of incense comes about and that an activation of the TRPV3 channel in the brain may play a certain role here was described in detail in a paper by A. Moussaieff in 2008.[24] Hallucinogens, which serve to intensify the experience of God, are also called **entheogens**. It is therefore quite conceivable that Zechariah also used entheogenic substances during the offering of the incense sacrifice, which favoured the occurrence of hallucinations.

Let's move on to the topic of **unfulfilled desire to have children**. In the absence of offspring, it used to be, and often still is, the "fault" of the woman who was infertile. It is only since artificial insemination has been offered to a broad public that the "normal population" has also come to realize that fertility problems can also be caused by **diseases of the man. However, this is only a realization** of recent times. Until the nineteenth century, infertility was always the woman's fault. Interestingly, fertility disorders are found more frequently in patients with schizophrenia than in healthy people. This has always been attributed to the drugs used to treat schizophrenics.[25] However, it has been shown that the fertility of schizophrenics is decreased overall.[26] Psychological stress alone associated with psychiatric illnesses, such as schizophrenia, can decrease male fertility,[27] presumably due to the stress-induced increase in **prolactin**, which can lead to decreased libido, erectile dysfunction and alteration of sperm composition. Patients with schizophrenia are more likely to show disturbances in sexual desire and function than is the case in the normal population.[28] So if we assume that Zechariah suffered from schizophrenia, then the childlessness, described in the Bible, is not entirely surprising. However, if one knows how much stress and psychological strain affect sexual function,[29] one can also understand that after an assurance (by an angel) of being able to have children, libido and sexual function can improve significantly, at least temporarily.

---

[24] Incensole acetate, an incense component, elicits psychoactivity by activating TRPV3 channels in the brain. Arieh Moussaieff, Neta Rimmerman, Tatiana Bregman, Alex Straiker, Christian C. Felder, Shai Shoham, Yoel Kashman, Susan M. Huang, Hyosang Lee, Esther Shohami, Ken Mackie, Michael J. Caterina, J. Michael Walker, Ester Fride, Raphael Mechoulam. FASEB J. 2008 Aug; 22(8): 3024–3034.

[25] Haddad, Peter M. and Angelika Wieck. "Antipsychotic-induced hyperprolactinaemia: mechanisms, clinical features and management." Drugs, vol. 64, no. 20, 2004, pp. 2291–2314. doi: https://doi.org/10.2165/00003495-200464200-00003).

[26] Bundy, H., et al. "A systematic review and meta-analysis of the fertility of patients with schizophrenia and their unaffected relatives." Acta Psychiatr. Scand. vol. 123, no. 2, Feb. 2011, pp. 98–106. doi: https://doi.org/10.1111/j.1600-0447.2010.01623.x.

[27] Nargund, Vinod H. "Effects of psychological stress on male fertility." Nat. Rev. Urol. vol. 12, July 2015, pp. 373–82. doi: https://doi.org/10.1038/nrurol.2015.112.

[28] Dumontaud, Marion, et al. "Sexual dysfunctions in schizophrenia: Beyond antipsychotics. A systematic review." Prog. Neuro-Psychopharmacol. Biol. Psychiatry, vol. 98, 2 Mar. 2020, p. 109804. doi: https://doi.org/10.1016/j.pnpbp.2019.109804.

[29] Herbert, Joe. "Sexuality, Stress, and the Chemical Architecture of the Brain." Annu. Rev. Sex Res., vol. 7, no. 1, 1 Mar. 1996, pp. 1–43. doi: https://doi.org/10.1080/10532528.1996.10559908.

Case report, infertility due to stress: You can also see this today in many young married couples with an unfulfilled desire to have children, who are under enormous stress. I remember a young couple who were both very stressed professionally and suffered from a constant lack of time. According to the recommendations of her gynaecologist, the woman determined her ovulation each time by a urine strip test. If the test was positive, she called her husband, and he had to come immediately and fulfil his marital duties. Through this ritual alone, the sexual behaviour of the two people was so disturbed that the desire for sex was permanently lost and offspring stubbornly failed to appear. Only after they were advised to stop testing and to have sex not according to the clock, but according to their individual desire, did the woman suddenly become "inexplicably" pregnant. This pregnancy came about solely because of the psychological relief! I was able to experience similar stories many times in the course of my medical practice. Stress and fear are extreme sex killers and also lead to biologically objective infertility. As soon as the pressure to have offspring is taken away, fertility works surprisingly often by itself, even if infertility has been "confirmed" by doctors for years. Anyone who has worked in a fertility clinic can confirm how much stress an unfulfilled desire to have children can mean for those affected. In a patriarchal society like 2000 years ago, where prestige and survival in old age was linked to having offspring, childlessness probably meant much more stress than it does today.

The "fertility of the ageing woman" is also not common, but still far from being a miracle. The fact that women in perimenopause can still become pregnant can be seen again and again even today.[30] How often does it happen that women after their "last" menstruation and supposed infertility, then still get pregnant. At that time such a thing was described as a "miracle"; today one would call it a caprice of nature because it does not occur frequently, but nevertheless it does occur.

Abstract: Schizophrenia with visual and auditory hallucinations (talking angel, ICD-10 R44.1 and R44.0), dialoguing voices (dialogue with the angel, ICD-10 F23.2), schizophrenic episode triggered by exposure to psychedelic substances (entheogenic smoke victim), mutism (inability to speak, ICD-10 F94.0, F20.5) and sterilitas matrimonii (unfulfilled desire to have children ICD-10 N97.4) probably in the context of subfertility in male schizophrenia and female perimenopause.

---

[30] Tarlatzis BC, Zepiridis L. Perimenopausal conception. Ann N Y Acad Sci. 2003 Nov;997:93–104. doi: https://doi.org/10.1196/annals.1290.011. PMID: 14644814.

What are entheogens? Entheogens are substances that are used in the context of ritual acts. In almost all cultures, such "mind-expanding" substances are used to intensify the "divine" experience. In the past, people prepared "smoke offerings" or took intoxicating drinks to achieve the most intense divine experience possible. Thus, many a ritual act became an "intoxicating feast."

Today, the Catholic Church still uses incense, which in high concentrations can have an antidepressant and anxiolytic effect, thus intensifying religious feelings. In other religions, fragrances in the form of incense sticks and scented oils are used as supposedly harmless substances to evoke pleasant feelings. These are actually psychedelic drugs with effects similar to narcotics. Even the wine used in the sacrifice of the Mass must originally have been regarded as an "intoxicant", but nowadays, it is drunk only in symbolic quantities.

1.3 The "Immaculate" Conception of Mary (The Miracle of the Virgin Birth)

1.3.1 Original Text (Luke 1:26–38; Matthew 1:18–25)

Birth of Jesus Foretold (Luke 1:26–38): 26 In the sixth month the angel Gabriel was sent from God to a city of Galilee named Nazareth, 27 to a virgin betrothed to a man whose name was Joseph, of the house of David. And the virgin's name was Mary. 28 And he came to her and said, "Greetings, O favoured one, the Lord is with you!" 29 But she was greatly troubled at the saying, and tried to discern what sort of greeting this might be. 30 And the angel said to her, "Do not be afraid, Mary, for you have found favour with God. 31 And behold, you will conceive in your womb and bear a son, and you shall call his name Jesus. 32 He will be great and will be called the Son of the Most High. And the Lord God will give to him the throne of his father David, 33 and he will reign over the house of Jacob forever, and of his kingdom there will be no end." 34 And Mary said to the angel, "How will this be, since I am a virgin?" 35 And the angel answered her, "The Holy Spirit will come upon you, and the power of the Most High will overshadow you; therefore the child to be born will be called holy—the Son of God. 36 And behold, your relative Elizabeth in her old age has also conceived a son, and this is the sixth month with her who was called barren. 37 For nothing will be impossible with God." 38 And Mary said, "Behold, I am the servant of the Lord; let it be to me according to your word." And the angel departed from her.

The Birth of Jesus Christ (Matthew 1:18–25): 18 Now, the birth of Jesus Christ took place in this way. When his mother Mary had been betrothed to Joseph, before they came together she was found to be with child from the Holy Spirit. 19 And her husband Joseph, being a just man and unwilling to put her to shame, resolved to divorce her quietly. 20 But as he considered these things, behold, an angel of the Lord appeared to him in a dream, saying, "Joseph, son of David, do not fear to take Mary as your wife, for that which is conceived in her is from the Holy Spirit. 21 She will bear a son, and you shall call his name Jesus, for he will save his people from their sins." 22 All this took place to fulfil what the Lord had spoken by the prophet: 23 "Behold, the virgin shall conceive and bear a son, and they shall call his name Immanuel" (which means, God with us). 24 When Joseph woke from sleep, he did as the angel of the Lord commanded him: he took his wife, 25 but knew her not until she had given birth to a son. And he called his name Jesus.

1.3.2 Description

The story of how Mary, the Mother of God, conceived her child is told as follows: At the time when Elizabeth, the wife of Zechariah was six months pregnant and was soon expecting her son, whom she was going to name John, a disaster happened. A close relative of hers, Mary, who was engaged to Joseph but not yet married, became pregnant. Since Mary was not yet married, she was threatened with a complete fall in social standing, if not death by stoning.

In the Bible, the following story is told as the "cause" of this apparently unplanned pregnancy: According to it, Mary became pregnant "by the Holy Spirit." The bearer of this "miraculous" message was once again the archangel Gabriel, who visited her and spoke to her in the following sense: "Do not be afraid, Mary, for you have found favour with God and you will conceive a son, to whom you shall give the name Jesus. The Holy Spirit will come upon you and will overshadow you. Your child will therefore also be called the Son of God".

Jesus is the name for "Son of the Most High" or, as the angel just said, "Son of God". This is the story of the "virgin" conception described in Luke's Gospel. A miraculous pregnancy that did not come about through conception by a man, but through the Holy Spirit.

1.3.3 Interpretation

The doctrine of the "**immaculate conception**" is to be distinguished from the "**virgin birth**". The "immaculate conception" is a dogma of the Catholic Church and simply states that Mary, as the "Mother of God", was preserved from any stain of original sin. In contrast, the virgin birth, is a procreation by God, that is, **parthenogenesis**.

The idea that a god unites with a human being and that descendants arise from this is not new and has already been handed down in many cultures. Greco-Roman mythology is full of demigods conceived by union of a human with a deity.[31] In Egyptian mythology, the pharaohs were conceived by union of the god Amun-Re

[31] Autoren der Wikimedia-Projekte. "Halbgott – Wikipedia." 22 Jan. 2004, de.wikipedia.org/w/index.php?title=Halbgott&oldid=216045474.

with the queen. Also, in Germanic[32] and Celtic mythology[33] there are "demigods" who were conceived by the union of a god and a human being.

The view that Mary was and remained a virgin did not emerge until around 200 A.D. It was created by the theologian Origenes (185–253 A.D.) and confirmed in the Synod of Rome (382 A.D.). Other proponents of this view were Peter of Alexandria, Epiphanus of Salamis, John Chrysostomos, St. Augustine and numerous other theologians.[34] In the Second Council of Constantinople, this doctrine was officially recognized in 553 A.D. and has been preserved until today.[35]

What really happened between Mary, the Mother of God and the Holy Spirit, we will never know. But the following interpretation possibilities seem to me in any case more probable than the **medically untenable hypothesis of a parthenogenesis, i.e. a virgin birth**:

> The **simplest explanation would be that of a translation error**. When the first German translation of the Septuagint was presented in January 2009, an article was found in the magazine "die Welt" a few days later, in which the translators stated the following translation error[36]:
>
> In the *ancient Septuagint*, Isaiah 7 reads, "Therefore the Lord Himself will give you a sign: Behold, the **virgin** (German Jungfrau) will be with child and bear a son. And you will give him the name Emanuel."
>
> In the *new German translation*, however, this passage reads, "Therefore the Lord Himself will give you a sign: behold, the **young woman** (German: junge Frau) will conceive and bear a son."

The term "**the virgin**" (Greek: parthenos, Latin: Virgo) has become "**the young woman**." In the Hebrew text the term was "almah" which means "young woman" and was mistakenly translated as "parthenos" (virgin).[37] This "small" translation error, however, would put the matter in a rather different light. In any case, in the third millennium, we can assume that the historical figure of Christ certainly did not come into being through conception without fertilization, but that the story of the "virgin" conception came into being much later. In any case, according to common sense, a **translation error** would be much more probable than a fertilization by the "Holy Spirit". The story of parthenogenesis, i.e. **divine fertilization**, would give the

---

32 Autoren der Wikimedia-Projekte. "Wieland der Schmied – Wikipedia." 12 Apr. 2003, de.wikipedia.org/w/index.php?title=Wieland_der_Schmied&oldid=214057285.

33 Autoren der Wikimedia-Projekte. "Keltische Mythologie – Wikipedia." 12 Sept. 2002, de.wikipedia.org/w/index.php?title=Keltische_Mythologie&oldid=215052185.

34 Autoren der Wikimedia-Projekte. "Immerwährende Jungfräulichkeit Marias – Wikipedia." 28 Apr. 2011, de.wikipedia.org/w/index.php?title=Immerw%C3%A4hrende_Jungfr%C3%A4ulichkeit_Marias&oldid=214929435.

35 "Konzile von Konstantinopel - Ökumenisches Heiligenlexikon." 10 Sept. 2020, www.heiligenlexikon.de/Glossar/Konzile_von_Konstantinopel.html.

36 Übersetzungsfehler machte Maria zur Jungfrau. Veröffentlicht am 28.01.2009. https://www.welt.de/kultur/article3100214/Uebersetzungsfehler-machte-Maria-zur-Jungfrau.html.

37 Thomsen, Hans Markus. "Bibelauslegung: Warum Maria wohl keine Jungfrau war." DIE WELT, 3 Oct. 2015, www.welt.de/wissenschaft/article2925511/Warum-Maria-wohl-keine-Jungfrau-war.html. [Why Mary was probably not a virgin].

Christian faith a divine "raison d'être", and for this one was apparently prepared to twist things a bit.

Another obvious explanation would be that Elizabeth wanted to help the young Mary and helped her with a story to escape social ostracism or even stoning. She herself had become pregnant by a "miracle" at an old age. An angel prophesied to her husband Zechariah that she could become pregnant after all, despite her advanced age and widely known infertility. **The story that one could miraculously become pregnant with the help of an angel was believed by all**. So what could be more obvious than to apply this story once again and thus save Mary's life. As a reminder, Mary was engaged but not yet allowed to marry, possibly because her fiancé Joseph did not yet have enough money to marry his beloved Mary. Apparently, she became pregnant during this time of waiting. One may assume that this was a catastrophe at that time and was possibly punished with death, but at least meant social ruin.

Elizabeth possibly not only helped her to spread this story and make it credible, but also invited her to her home for the time of pregnancy. More than that, if Elizabeth was foretold by Zechariah during the apparition that her son (John the Baptist), would be the forerunner of the longed-for Messiah, then the next "miraculous" conception must be the Messiah.

Joseph, was torn whether to leave his fiancée, Mary or stay with her. He did like her, but the honour of his family was at stake. Here, too, the "apparition" of an angel was able to remedy the situation and resolve the conflict. Since everyone already believed in the angel's story of Elizabeth, Joseph was able to save the honour of his family through the angel's command on the one hand, and on the other hand, he was able to follow his sense of responsibility and stand by his fiancée Mary. So he decided to stay with her after all. Admittedly, under these circumstances, it did not make sense to stay in the hometown. Perhaps that is why Mary and Joseph were happy to move away. In any case, the census of the emperor Augustus was certainly a welcome reason to suddenly have to leave the hometown.

Of course, nobody can say whether this story really happened like this or not, but it is at any rate more credible and much more probable than a parthenogenesis.

The Consequences of a Translation Error

The Septuagint is the oldest continuous translation of the Hebrew-Aramaic Bible into the Greek language of the time. The translation was produced from about 250 B.C. to A.D. 100, primarily in Alexandria. Originally, the term Septuagint referred to the translation of the Torah (the five books of Moses). Later, the term was expanded, primarily by Christians, to include the Greek versions of the Old Testament. In this later form, the Septuagint included all the Greek-translated books of the Hebrew Bible. The Septuagint survives today as the Christian scriptural tradition in Greek. Judaism has rejected the Septuagint since ancient times, although it was initially given credence.[38] When the first German translation was presented a few years ago, it delivered a few surprises. The idea of the virgin conception apparently came into the world with the Septuagint. For the "young woman" in Hebrew suddenly becomes "virgin" in Greek translation. This translation error may have been very congenial to the ecclesiastical moral ideas of late antiquity and the Middle Ages.

Abstract: *Translation error* or *white lie* with which Elizabeth saved the life of Mary, who was close to her. One can choose.

1.4 The Wedding at Cana (The Transformation of Water into Wine)

1.4.1 Original Text (John 2:1–12)

The Wedding at Cana (John 2:1–12): 1 On the third day there was a wedding at Cana in Galilee, and the mother of Jesus was there. 2 Jesus also was invited to the wedding with his disciples. 3 When the wine ran out, the mother of Jesus said to him, "They have no wine." 4 And Jesus said to her, "Woman, what does this have to do with me? My hour has not yet come." 5 His mother said to the servants, "Do whatever he tells you." 6 Now there were six stone water jars there for the Jewish rites of purification, each holding twenty or thirty gallons. 7 Jesus said to the servants, "Fill the jars with water." And they filled them up to the brim. 8 And he said to them, "Now draw some out and take it to the master of the feast." So they took it. 9 When the master of the feast tasted the water now become wine, and did not know where it came from (though the servants who had drawn the water knew), the master of the feast called the bridegroom 10 and said to him, "Everyone serves the good wine first, and when people have drunk freely, then the poor wine. But you have kept the good wine until now." 11 This, the first of his signs, Jesus did at Cana in Galilee, and manifested his glory. And his disciples believed in him. 12 After this he went down to Capernaum, with his mother and his brothers and his disciples, and they stayed there for a few days.

1.4.2 Description and Interpretation

Jesus was invited with his family to a wedding with good friends. The guests drank so much that the wine threatened to run out. Anyone who has ever experienced an oriental wedding can well imagine that it may have been quite boozy and merry. Weddings are still so important for the Oriental that it is common to go into debt in order to offer the invited guests an "appropriate" celebration. It would be a great

[38] Autoren der Wikimedia-Projekte. "Septuaginta – Wikipedia." 10 Oct. 2002, de.wikipedia.org/w/index.php?title=Septuaginta&oldid=217241519.

embarrassment for a host if the wine ran out. No host would want to be considered stingy, as this would be associated with a loss of his social standing. Mary apparently recognized in time the problem that there might not be enough wine left and asked her son Jesus to remedy the situation.

If there was not enough wine and right next to the wine jugs there were large water jugs, what was more obvious than to water down the wine. The already drunken guests—obviously more wine was drunk than was usual—would certainly not notice this.

But why was the diluted wine even considered better? It is known that the Romans at that time sweetened the wine with lead acetate, because otherwise it tasted sour.[39] However, only the upper class of rich Romans could afford this sweetened wine. One can assume therefore that the normal wine tasted rather sour in those days. The common people especially could not afford the sweetened wine like the wealthy Roman upper class. Therefore, they had to make do with the sour wine. That this social difference in the consumption of wine actually existed at that time can be seen from excavations. Archaeologists distinguish the bones of Roman legionaries and Roman officers by the lead content in the bones. The officers could afford the expensive wine sweetened with lead acetate, while the legionaries had to settle for the sour wine. Therefore, the bones of Roman officers have a higher lead content than the bones of the foot soldiers and can be distinguished easily.[40]

With the Jews it will not have been much different, and they will have had to be content with the cheap sour wine. In the story told above, it is also confirmed that the wine served first did not taste so good, possibly because it was too sour. And how to improve the sour taste of the wine? Simply by adding water to it! The wine increases in a "miraculous way" and it "tastes even better". The already quite tipsy wedding party might not have really noticed the swindle. One would call such behaviour a "white lie" or "politeness swindle". A lie of courtesy is defined as: "an untrue statement that serves to protect social relations and has more the function of a polite gesture".[41]

Abstract: Diluting wine with water, a saving grace that is most likely to be interpreted as a "politeness swindle".

[39] Eisinger J. Lead and wine. Eberhard Gockel and the colica Pictonum. Med Hist. 1982 Jul;26(3):279–302. doi: https://doi.org/10.1017/s0025727300041508. PMID: 6750289; PMCID: PMC1139187.

[40] Personal communication of an archeologist.

[41] Definition "Höflichkeitslüge – Wiktionary." 7 Nov. 2021, de.wiktionary.org/wiki/H%C3%B6flichkeitsl%C3%BCge.

1.5 Jesus Heals an Official's Son (Healing of a Civil Servant's Son in Cana)

1.5.1 Original Text (John 4:46–54)

Jesus Heals an Official's Son (John 4:46–54): 46 So he came again to Cana in Galilee, where he had made the water wine. And at Capernaum there was an official whose son was ill. 47 When this man heard that Jesus had come from Judea to Galilee, he went to him and asked him to come down and heal his son, for he was at the point of death. 48 So Jesus said to him, "Unless you see signs and wonders you will not believe." 49 The official said to him, "Sir, come down before my child dies." 50 Jesus said to him, "Go; your son will live." The man believed the word that Jesus spoke to him and went on his way. 51 As he was going down, his servants met him and told him that his son was recovering. 52 So he asked them the hour when he began to get better, and they said to him, "Yesterday at the seventh hour the fever left him." 53 The father knew that was the hour when Jesus had said to him, "Your son will live." And he himself believed, and all his household. 54 This was now the second sign that Jesus did when he had come from Judea to Galilee.

1.5.2 Description and Interpretation

Jesus left Judea and returned to Galilee. Since the miraculous transformation of water into wine, his reputation as a "miracle worker" preceded him. A high official, whose son lay sick at home with a fever, hastened to meet Jesus to ask him to heal his dying son. Jesus did not respond to the official's request at all, but simply replied, "Your son is alive," thus making no move to enter the official's home. The royal official went home strengthened by the faith that his son would be restored to health. Even before he reached his home, his servants came to meet him and told him that his son had recovered. The healing apparently took place at the very hour when Jesus told him that his son would survive and not die.

Jesus knew, or at least felt, that his "effect" depended essentially on whether people believed in him. That is why he moved away from his home. He went back to the area where he already had a "good reputation", namely to Galilee. There he had already been successful once, when he had changed "water into wine". The fact that one is never so recognized where one grew up is a well-known phenomenon. It is not for nothing that the saying from the Bible "**The prophet counts for nothing in his own country**" (according to Luke 4:24) has survived for millennia. Jesus obviously experienced that in his hometown, nobody really wanted to believe in him. In Galilee, it was different. Having arrived there, Jesus soon had the opportunity to perform "miracles". An official of the king, obviously an influential person, heard about his ability to perform miracles. He rushed to him, told of his "dying" son, and asked Jesus to come to his house. Apparently, the son had a fever (John 4:52).

The most common cause of fever is infection, but there is also **psychogenic fever**, which occurs mainly in young or mentally unstable people. In this case, the stress hormone adrenaline is released as part of a stress reaction. This stimulates, among other things, ß3 receptors on the cells of the brown adipose tissue. This leads to what is known as "**beta-3 adrenoreceptor-mediated thermogenesis**".[42] When help approaches or a solution to the problem is in sight, the stress reaction stops. The adrenaline level drops and the fever decreases. The typical characteristic of psychogenic fever is the fever, subsiding as soon as help is in sight. In this case, one can assume a spontaneous healing, which occurred after the father of the sick son left the house to get help from a "miracle healer".

The Bible also states that the healing of the sick son occurred just at the time when Jesus told the father that his son was not dying ("Go; your son will live!", John 4:50). From this synchronicity, a miraculous healing is inferred. **Synchronicity** refers to "temporally correlated events that are not linked by a causal relationship, but are perceived and interpreted as connected, related to each other."[43] Apart from the fact that at that time the determination of temporal coincidences was not even possible, it must be pointed out that coincidences are not an expression of causality. With temporally coinciding events the large danger of a false conclusion exists, also called **pseudo causality**, a problem with which the philosophers have concerned themselves already for a long time: "Cum hoc non est propter hoc", "with this" does not mean "therefore".[44] Obviously, it lies in the nature of humans to see temporally coinciding events also as causally connected events. This phenomenon is called causal attribution.[45] In this case, there is an external causal attribution, but certainly no causality.

Let us return to the "dying" son: If he had a quite banal infection with chills and poor general condition, then the normal course of an infection would be that there is initially a fever and this fever spontaneously subsides again. This is the normal course of an infection. In the present case, however, a psychogenic fever is more likely, especially since the reduction in fever coincided with the prospect of help.

Abstract: Normal spontaneous recovery after febrile infection (ICD-10 R50.88) or psychogenic fever (ICD-10 R50.-). Temporal coincidence of two events (synchronicity) with apparent causality.

---

[42] Oka T. Psychogenic fever: how psychological stress affects body temperature in the clinical population. Temperature (Austin). 2015 Jun 3;2(3):368–78. doi: https://doi.org/10.1080/23328940.2015.1056907. PMID: 27227051; PMCID: PMC4843908.

[43] Autoren der Wikimedia-Projekte. "Synchronizität – Wikipedia." 7 Mar. 2004, de.wikipedia.org/w/index.php?title=Synchronizit%C3%A4t&oldid=216640960.

[44] Autoren der Wikimedia-Projekte. "Cum hoc ergo propter hoc – Wikipedia." 8 Apr. 2005, de.wikipedia.org/w/index.php?title=Cum_hoc_ergo_propter_hoc&oldid=217267361.

[45] Weiner B. Attribution theory and attributional therapy: some theoretical observations and suggestions. Br J Clin Psychol. 1988 Feb;27(1):99–104. doi: https://doi.org/10.1111/j.2044-8260.1988.tb00757.x. PMID: 3355911.

1.6 The Healing at the Pool on the Sabbath (Healing of the Paralysed Man)

1.6.1 Original Text (John 5:1–17)

The Healing at the Pool on the Sabbath (John 5:1–17): 1 After this there was a feast of the Jews, and Jesus went up to Jerusalem. 2 Now there is in Jerusalem by the Sheep Gate a pool, in Aramaic called Bethesda, which has five roofed colonnades. 3 In these lay a multitude of invalids—blind, lame, and paralysed. 5 One man was there who had been an invalid for thirty-eight years. 6 When Jesus saw him lying there and knew that he had already been there a long time, he said to him, "Do you want to be healed?" 7 The sick man answered him, "Sir, I have no one to put me into the pool when the water is stirred up, and while I am going another steps down before me." 8 Jesus said to him, "Get up, take up your bed, and walk." 9 And at once the man was healed, and he took up his bed and walked. Now, that day was the Sabbath. 10 So the Jews said to the man who had been healed, "It is the Sabbath, and it is not lawful for you to take up your bed." 11 But he answered them, "The man who healed me, that man said to me, 'Take up your bed, and walk.'" 12 They asked him, "Who is the man who said to you, 'Take up your bed and walk'?" 13 Now the man who had been healed did not know who it was, for Jesus had withdrawn, as there was a crowd in the place. 14 Afterward, Jesus found him in the temple and said to him, "See, you are well! Sin no more, that nothing worse may happen to you." 15 The man went away and told the Jews that it was Jesus who had healed him. 16 And this was why the Jews were persecuting Jesus, because he was doing these things on the Sabbath. 17 But Jesus answered them, "My Father is working until now, and I am working."

1.6.2 Description and Interpretation

Near Jerusalem, there was a pond with the name "Bethesda", which was said to have healing properties. Therefore, five columned halls had been built there, and many sick people gathered there, waiting to be carried into the water by their relatives or other people. They hoped to be healed by it.

There was also a man lying there who had been sick for 38 years. Jesus saw him and asked him if he wanted to get well again. The sick man replied that he had no one to carry him into the water. Every time he drags himself to the water, someone else goes in before him, so he cannot enter the water. Thus, he had no chance of being healed. After the man complained to Jesus about his suffering, Jesus said to him, "Get up, take up your bed, and walk!". Thereupon, the man got up and apparently walked away healed.

Even today we know of spas where people go on pilgrimage hoping for a miraculous healing. Lourdes is one of the most famous places to which such healing powers are attributed. But also place names like Heiligwasser, Heiligbrunn (Heilbronn) etc. point to the belief of people that diseases could be cured by "holy water".

What happened at the pond in Bethesda might have been no different. If Jesus had wanted to heal all sick people, it would have been very likely that he would have been unsuccessful. Probably he chose a suitable "victim" for his miracle work. A person who was obviously alone, "for he had no one to help him plunge into the healing waters". Someone who evidently could still walk, but apparently put himself on the back burner because he couldn't push through when others pushed into the water in front of him. A person who had been "apologizing for being alive" for many years,[46] a person who had no confidence in himself.[47] One of the problems with people with low self-esteem is that they experience, just by their help-seeking behaviour, aversion from the people whose help they seek.[48] Thus, they get more and more sidelined and have little prospect that someone comes to help them.

This is exactly the type of man with whom one may expect success **offering attention** and **by suggestive commands**. The Bible says that he was still able to walk, even if not so well (John 5:7). But he could not prevail. Since the walking difficulties had already existed for 38 years, one can assume that it was a **psychogenic paralysis of infancy or adolescence**.[49]

An "unstable" person can be "cured" just by strengthening his self-confidence, empowering him again and giving him more backbone, by standing before him as a miracle worker and giving the command "Get up, take your bed and walk". Jesus had often used the command form to miraculously heal people who were inhibiting themselves. This is exactly what happened.

By 1927 it had already been described how one can heal merely by suggestive commands.[50] It is also known today that decreased self-esteem is associated with a disturbance of the pituitary-adrenal axis (stress hormone production).[51] The worse one feels, the lower the ability to mobilize stress hormones in the adrenal gland and the lower the production of beta-endorphins. The lack of these hormones, however, in turn causes people to feel bad. A vicious circle, which Jesus apparently broke here with a "**suggestive command**". Hormone production is stimulated again, the "spirits of life" return and one experiences strength, self-confidence and a sense of vitality. Nothing else is done today by psychologists, psychotherapists, hypnotherapists, coaches, etc., and apparently they do not make a bad living at it.

---

[46] Castro NB, Lopes MVO, Monteiro ARM. Low Chronic Self-Esteem and Low Situational Self-Esteem: a literature review. Rev Bras Enferm. 2020 Feb 10;73(1):e20180004. English, Portuguese. doi: https://doi.org/10.1590/0034-7167-2018-0004. PMID: 32049223.

[47] Oney E, Oksuzoglu-Guven G. Confidence: a critical review of the literature and an alternative perspective for general and specific self-confidence. Psychol Rep. 2015 Feb;116(1):149–63. doi: https://doi.org/10.2466/07.PR0.116k14w0. Epub 2015 Jan 26. PMID: 25621670.

[48] Don BP, Girme YU, Hammond MD. Low Self-Esteem Predicts Indirect Support Seeking and Its Relationship Consequences in Intimate Relationships. Pers Soc Psychol Bull. 2019 Jul;45(7):1028–1041. doi: https://doi.org/10.1177/0146167218802837. Epub 2018 Nov 22. PMID: 30465478.

[49] Nowak M. Psychogene Lähmungen im Kindes- und Jugendalter [Psychogenic paralysis in childhood and adolescence]. Z Kinder Jugendpsychiatr Psychother. 2002 Aug;30(3):199–210. German. doi: https://doi.org/10.1024//1422-4917.30.3.199. PMID: 12227222.

[50] Bloch, Bruno. "Über die Heilung der Warzen durch Suggestion." Klin. Wochenschr., vol. 6, no. 49, 1 Dec. 1927, pp. 2320–5. doi: https://doi.org/10.1007/BF01726552.

[51] Zorrilla EP, DeRubeis RJ, Redei E.: Psychoneuroendocrinology. 1995;20(6):591–601. High self-esteem, hardiness and affective stability are associated with higher basal pituitary-adrenal hormone levels. PMID:8584600.

Psychogenic paralyses can occur as monopareses, hemipareses, parapareses or tetrapareses. Differentiation from simulation and aggravation is difficult in paralyses.[52] Psychogenic paralyses can be triggered by conflicts and stress, but especially after traumatic stress. If a psychogenic paralysis persists for years, regression (atrophy) of the musculature usually also occurs. An overview of psychogenic movement disorders can be found in an article by S. Kranick 2011.[53]

Abstract: Nowadays, the diagnosis would be: **dissociative disorder (ICD-10 F44) with paralysis symptoms (ICD-10 F54), cure by suggestive command**.

1.7 Jesus Calls the First Disciples (The Wonderful Fishing)

1.7.1 Original Text (Luke 5:1–11)

Jesus Calls the First Disciples (Luke 5:1–11): 1 On one occasion, while the crowd was
pressing in on him to hear the word of God, he was standing by the lake of Gennesaret, 2
and he saw two boats by the lake, but the fishermen had gone out of them and were washing
their nets. 3 Getting into one of the boats, which was Simon's, he asked him to put out a
little from the land. And he sat down and taught the people from the boat. 4 And when he
had finished speaking, he said to Simon, "Put out into the deep and let down your nets for a
catch." 5 And Simon answered, "Master, we toiled all night and took nothing! But at your
word, I will let down the nets." 6 And when they had done this, they enclosed a large number
of fish, and their nets were breaking. 7 They signaled to their partners in the other boat to
come and help them. And they came and filled both the boats, so that they began to sink. 8
But when Simon Peter saw it, he fell down at Jesus' knees, saying, "Depart from me, for I
am a sinful man, O Lord." 9 For he and all who were with him were astonished at the catch
of fish that they had taken, 10 and so also were James and John, sons of Zebedee, who were
partners with Simon. And Jesus said to Simon, "Do not be afraid; from now on you will be
catching men." 11 And when they had brought their boats to land, they left everything and
followed him.

1.7.2 Description and Interpretation

Jesus wanted to give a speech at the Sea of Galilee. After the crowd had become very large and Jesus was pressed to preach the word of God, he let Peter take him in his fishing boat a little way from land. From there, Jesus then gave his speech. When he had finished and Peter took him back to land, Jesus told Peter to go out on the lake once more and cast his nets in the **deep** water. Peter did not find this to be a very reasonable thing to do, having fished all night and caught nothing. To an experienced

[52] Communications, Ebcont. "Psychogene Lähmung." 21 July 2021, eref.thieme.de/cockpits/0/0/coNeuro00352/0.

[53] Kranick, Sarah M., et al. "Psychogenic Movement Disorders and Motor Conversion: A Roadmap for Collaboration Between Neurology and Psychiatry." Psychosomatics, vol. 52, no. 2, 1 Mar. 2011, pp. 109–16. doi: https://doi.org/10.1016/j.psym.2010.12.017.

fisherman, everything spoke against catching anything during the day. Nevertheless, he went out because Jesus had told him to. **Amazingly, they caught so many fish in the deep water that he not only filled his own boat with fish, but had to get a second boat to retrieve all the fish from the nets**. Peter was so overwhelmed by this unusual catch of fish that he threw himself at Jesus' feet.

Probably the fish caught was mainly the so-called "Peter's fish" (Acanthobrama terraesanctae) which belongs to the carp family (Cyprinidae).[54] These belong to the "peaceful fish", are very common in the Sea of Galilee and are caught mainly at dusk or at night with the net. During daylight hours, they retreat from the surface to avoid being seen easily by predatory fish. However, when the weather turns cloudy or wind comes up, this can change quickly and one can easily have good catches during the day. Jesus gave the recommendation, "**Go out where it is deep and cast your nets for a catch!**". With this recommendation, the schools of fish that were not quite at the surface during daylight could be caught well.

The essence of this story, however, is the fact that **Jesus encouraged the apostle Peter and his helpers** to go out for another catch. **Even if the external circumstances speak against it, one should not give up**. Peter, as an experienced fisherman, will not have been so stupid as to go to the same fishing grounds where he had already fished unsuccessfully during the night. So he sought out another "unusual place," deep waters, and lo and behold, he found what he was looking for and caught more fish than usual. **The message here is not so much the miracle of a successful fish catch as the fact that one should not give up in the face of failure**. There are numerous books about the effect of motivation and perseverance despite existing adversities, and a whole branch of science of motivation research.

Abstract: Success through motivation and perseverance despite adversity (motivation research).

1.8 Jesus Heals a Man with an Unclean Spirit (Exorcism of Demons in the Synagogue of Capernaum)

1.8.1 Original Text of the Bible (Luke 4:31–41; Mark 1:21–28)

Jesus Heals a Man with an Unclean Demon (Luke 4:31–41): 31 And he went down to Capernaum, a city of Galilee. And he was teaching them on the Sabbath, 32 and they were astonished at his teaching, for his word possessed authority. 33 And in the synagogue there was a man who had the spirit of an unclean demon, and he cried out with a loud voice, 34 "Ha! What have you to do with us, Jesus of Nazareth? Have you come to destroy us? I know who you are—the Holy One of God." 35 But Jesus rebuked him, saying, "Be silent and come out of him!" And when the demon had thrown him down in their midst, he came out of him,

[54] Contributors to Wikimedia projects. "Acanthobrama terraesanctae - Wikipedia." 15 Nov. 2021, en.wikipedia.org/w/index.php?title=Acanthobrama_terraesanctae&oldid=1055296245.

having done him no harm. 36 And they were all amazed and said to one another, "What is this word? For with authority and power he commands the unclean spirits, and they come out!" 37 And reports about him went out into every place in the surrounding region.

Jesus Heals a Man with an Unclean Spirit (Mark 1:21–28): 21 And they went into Capernaum, and immediately on the Sabbath he entered the synagogue and was teaching. 22 And they were astonished at his teaching, for he taught them as one who had authority, and not as the scribes. 23 And immediately there was in their synagogue a man with an unclean spirit. And he cried out, 24 "What have you to do with us, Jesus of Nazareth? Have you come to destroy us? I know who you are—the Holy One of God." 25 But Jesus rebuked him, saying, "Be silent, and come out of him!" 26 And the unclean spirit, convulsing him and crying out with a loud voice, came out of him. 27 And they were all amazed, so that they questioned among themselves, saying, "What is this? A new teaching with authority! He commands even the unclean spirits, and they obey him." 28 And at once his fame spread everywhere throughout all the surrounding region of Galilee.

1.8.2 Description and Interpretation

This story is about Jesus presenting his views in the synagogue of Capernaum. He spoke with such conviction that resistance arose among the audience, at least among the very conservative Jews. One of the listeners apparently felt personally attacked by the new teachings and "snapped." It seems that this man was known to behave "peculiarly" again and again, because it says in the Bible "that he was possessed by an unclean spirit." Today, such a person would be called a "freak" or "short-tempered." So an incident occurred: the listener shouted, "What have we to do with you, Jesus of Nazareth? Have you come to destroy us?" Jesus did not respond with gentlemanly restraint, but apparently shouted back that he should be silent. Well knowing that this man was considered "possessed", he added to the "command to be silent" the command, "and leave him". Saying this, he alluded to the "evil spirit" which supposedly sat in the listener. The person concerned threw himself to the ground in a manner similar to an irascible child, screamed some more, and then calmed down again without anything else happening as a result. This embarrassing incident caused the whole audience to be quite startled. The fact that the "possessed one" calmed down again after this incident apparently led to Jesus being perceived as someone who had the power to "conquer evil spirits."

Outbursts of rage occur all the time.[55] Especially people with psychiatric diseases have such impulse control losses.[56] If they occur more often, psychiatrists speak of

[55] Fariba K, Gokarakonda SB. Impulse Control Disorders. 2021 Aug 30. In: StatPearls [Internet]. Treasure Island (FL): StatPearls Publishing; 2021 Jan. PMID: 32965950.

[56] Silva B, Canas-Simião H, Cavanna AE. Neuropsychiatric Aspects of Impulse Control Disorders. Psychiatr Clin North Am. 2020 Jun;43(2):249–262. doi: https://doi.org/10.1016/j.psc.2020.02.001. Epub 2020 Apr 8. PMID: 32439020.

"intermittent explosive disorder".[57] In common parlance, one speaks of pathological irascibility. In history, there are many known cases of impulse control disorders: Moses, for example, famously slew an overseer in a fit of rage. Many despots are reported to have had recurrent outbursts of rage. It is said of a recent state President that there was a specific man in the White House (so-called "music man") whose job it was to calm his boss down again when he threw a tantrum.[58] A top model was convicted of a temper tantrum in which she spat at and kicked a police officer with her boot.[59] The list of celebrity temper tantrums could go on and on. If one enters the search word "slain" in the Bible, one lands 87 hits, places in which someone was slain in the Old Testament.[60] In any case, it should show that such states of an "intermittent explosive disorder" are not rare.

According to today's opinion, such impulsive aggressions (outbursts of rage, pathological irascibility, intermittent explosive disorder) are not an expression of a personality disorder, but are due to a disturbed development of the emotional brain. MRI studies showed that the more pronounced the aggressive behaviour, the less the frontolimbic gray matter.[61] That is, the stronger the pathological irascibility, the smaller the volume of the 'emotional' brain area.[62] Possibly, such behaviour is triggered by infections with the parasite Toxoplasma gondii.[63] In any case, it is easy to imagine that in the past, **people with intermittent aggression disorder were considered 'possessed'. Episodes of intermittent explosive disorder are self-limited and usually resolve spontaneously**. However, punishment rage episodes can be terminated prematurely.[64] But in these cases there is usually a renewed "barrage of anger." Jesus won the battle of words, actually made the "possessed one" ridiculous in front

---

[57] Fanning JR, Coleman M, Lee R, Coccaro EF. Subtypes of aggression in intermittent explosive disorder. J Psychiatr Res. 2019 Feb;109:164-172. doi: https://doi.org/10.1016/j.jpsychires.2018.10.013. Epub 2018 Oct 19. PMID: 30551023; PMCID: PMC6699742.

[58] Orf. at. "Ex-Sprecherin: „Musik-Mann" sollte N.N. beruhigen." News.ORF, 28 Sept. 2021, orf.at/stories/3230397.

[59] Dawar, Anil. "N.N. pleads guilty to assaulting airport police." the Guardian, 2 July 2018, www.theguardian.com/uk/2008/jun/20/ukcrime.fashion.

[60] ""erschlagen" | Einheitsübersetzung 2016: ERF Bibleserver." 22 Nov. 2021, www.bibleserver.com/search/EU/erschlagen.

[61] Coccaro EF, Fitzgerald DA, Lee R, McCloskey M, Phan KL. Frontolimbic Morphometric Abnormalities in Intermittent Explosive Disorder and Aggression. Biol Psychiatry Cogn Neurosci Neuroimaging. 2016 Jan;1(1):32–38. doi: https://doi.org/10.1016/j.bpsc.2015.09.006. Epub 2015 Oct 14. PMID: 29560894.

[62] Coccaro EF, Lee R, McCloskey M, Csernansky JG, Wang L. Morphometric analysis of amygdala and hippocampus shape in impulsively aggressive and healthy control subjects. J Psychiatr Res. 2015 Oct;69:80–6. doi: https://doi.org/10.1016/j.jpsychires.2015.07.009. Epub 2015 Jul 13. PMID: 26343598; PMCID: PMC5978418.

[63] Sugden K, Moffitt TE, Pinto L, Poulton R, Williams BS, Caspi A. Is Toxoplasma Gondii Infection Related to Brain and Behavior Impairments in Humans? Evidence from a Population-Representative Birth Cohort. PLoS One. 2016 Feb 17;11(2):e0148435. doi: https://doi.org/10.1371/journal.pone.0148435. PMID: 26886853; PMCID: PMC4757034.

[64] Puhalla AA, Ammerman BA, Uyeji LL, Berman ME, McCloskey MS. Negative urgency and reward/punishment sensitivity in intermittent explosive disorder. J Affect Disord. 2016 Sep 1;201:8–14. doi: https://doi.org/10.1016/j.jad.2016.04.045. Epub 2016 Apr 27. PMID: 27155024.

of the congregation, and thus punished him in a way. Just as a small child throws itself on the ground when it is no longer able to successfully defend itself, so did this "possessed" man. The community apparently interpreted this peculiar behaviour to mean that the evil spirit had left the body.

Abstract: Intermittent explosive disorder (ICD-10 F63.8), aggressive episode with spontaneous resolution.

In the same chapter, the **miraculous healing of Peter's mother-in-law** is mentioned in a subordinate clause. This case is described in the next chapter. In the synagogue, at any rate, Jesus had been able to gain authority among his followers after he successfully ended a war of words in his favour with a loud-mouthed orthodox Jew. This incident strengthened not only his followers' faith, but also the wider public's faith in his abilities.

1.9 Fever of Peter's Mother-in-Law in Capernaum. (Jesus Heals Many)

1.9.1 Original Text (Luke 4:38–39; Mark 1:29–31; Matthew 8:14–15)

Jesus Heals Many (Luke 4:38–39): 38 And he arose and left the synagogue and entered Simon's house. Now Simon's mother-in-law was ill with a high fever, and they appealed to him on her behalf. 39 And he stood over her and rebuked the fever, and it left her, and immediately she rose and began to serve them. 40 Now when the sun was setting, all those who had any who were sick with various diseases brought them to him, and he laid his hands on every one of them and healed them. 41 And demons also came out of many, crying, "You are the Son of God!" But he rebuked them and would not allow them to speak, because they knew that he was the Christ.

Jesus Heals Many (Mark 1:29–31): 29 And immediately he[7] left the synagogue and entered the house of Simon and Andrew, with James and John. 30 Now Simon's mother-in-law lay ill with a fever, and immediately they told him about her. 31 And he came and took her by the hand and lifted her up, and the fever left her, and she began to serve them.

Jesus Heals Many (Matthew 8:14–15): 14 And when Jesus entered Peter's house, he saw his mother-in-law lying sick with a fever. 15 He touched her hand, and the fever left her, and she rose and began to serve him.

1.9.2 Description and Interpretation

Following the talk in the synagogue and after "successfully casting out a demon," Jesus left the synagogue and was invited by Simon Peter to his home. Apparently, after this episode, he enjoyed even more prestige and authority than before. With the others, he went to the house of Simon and his family, where Simon's mother-in-law had been complaining about fever for some time. The sick mother-in-law's relatives told her about the incident in the synagogue. Thus, of course, Jesus had gained much authority over Simon's mother-in-law. Equipped with this authority, Jesus now approached the sick woman, took her hand and "commanded" her to get up. The fever that had been with her for a long time suddenly left her as if by a miracle, and she got up and was able to perform her domestic duties and entertain the guests.

Fevers that can be treated so quickly by authoritative behaviour meet the criteria for a "psychogenic fever." This involves temperatures between 37.5 and 38.0 °C, in rare cases up to 41 °C[65]. The patients mostly show a cool and pale facial skin.[66] Triggers for this are emotional conflicts as well as anxiety, restlessness, and states of tension.[67]

Abstract: Psychogenic fever (ICD-10 F45 or ICD-10 R50.88).

1.10 Healing the Masses

1.10.1 Original Text of the Bible (Luke 4:40–41, Mark 1:32–34)

Jesus Heals Many (Luke 4:40–41): 38 And he arose and left the synagogue and entered Simon's house. Now Simon's mother-in-law was ill with a high fever, and they appealed to him on her behalf. 39 And he stood over her and rebuked the fever, and it left her, and immediately she rose and began to serve them. 40 Now when the sun was setting, all those who had any who were sick with various diseases brought them to him, and he laid his hands on every one of them and healed them. 41 And demons also came out of many, crying, "You are the Son of God!" But he rebuked them and would not allow them to speak, because they knew that he was the Christ.

Jesus Heals Many (Mark 1:32–34): That evening at sundown they brought to him all who were sick or oppressed by demons. 33 And the whole city was gathered together at the door. 34 And he healed many who were sick with various diseases, and cast out many demons. And he would not permit the demons to speak, because they knew him.

[65] Olivier B. Psychogenic fever, functional fever, or psychogenic hyperthermia? Temperature (Austin). 2015 Aug 3;2(3):324–5. doi: https://doi.org/10.1080/23328940.2015.1071701. PMID: 27227037; PMCID: PMC4843918.

[66] Oka, Takakazu and Kae Oka. "Mechanisms of Psychogenic Fever." Adv. Neuroimmune Biol., vol. 3, no. 1, 1 Jan. 2012, pp. 3–17. doi: https://doi.org/10.3233/NIB-2012-011030.

[67] Oka, Takakazu. "Handbook of Clinical Neurology." Stress-induced hyperthermia and hypothermia. Elsevier, 1 Jan. 2018, pp. 599–621. doi: https://doi.org/10.1016/B978-0-444-64074-1.00035-5.

1.10.2 Description and Interpretation

After Jesus "cast out a demon" in the synagogue and miraculously delivered Simon's mother-in-law from her fever, word of these miraculous healings spread throughout the village. People brought all kinds of sick and possessed people to him so that he could heal them. It is not known which diseases these were, the diseases were not described in the Bible, either. Jesus also had a lot of success here, so that one can assume psychosomatic diseases. Especially, somatoform disorders can be miraculously cured by "the physician as a medicine" alone.[68] The psychological effects of doctors were described very precisely by Balint.[69] With the term "The physician as a medicine" he explains how pain and numerous other complaints can be treated successfully, without drug therapy, just by the attention of the doctor. His methods are still used today.[70]

Who does not know the phenomenon that one goes to the dentist because of toothache and when the competent help is in reach, the toothache is gone? Yes, one can not even say which tooth exactly had hurt. Or one goes to the doctor because of a complaint like itching, pain, fever, rash etc. and as soon one is in the doctor's office and the help in prospect, it is embarrassing for the patient, because all complaints are **as if "gone"**. Every doctor knows such situations, but would never call it a miracle cure. **The prospect of healing is often enough for decisive healing processes to be spontaneously initiated.**[71] Psychologists refer to this phenomenon as "**self-fulfilling prophecy**", physicians as **placebo effect.**[72] In medicine, the placebo effect is the occurrence of a therapeutic effect through sham treatments, especially after administration of sham preparations such as tablets without active ingredients, so-called **placebos**. The **laying on of hands** is one of the oldest therapeutic procedures. It is often so effective that in the German language one does not speak of therapy but of treatment ("be-handeln"). The word for treatment ("be-handeln") contains the word "hand".

Abstract: Placebo effect, self-fulfilling prophecy, treatment by laying on of hands.

---

[68] Hoppen, Thomas and Marcel Kraemer. "Was die "Droge" Arzt bewirken kann." Pädiatrie, vol. 32, no. 6, 1 Dec. 2020, p. 48. doi: https://doi.org/10.1007/s15014-020-2459-x.

[69] Main TF. Michael Balint and his contributions. Psychiatry Med. 1972 Oct;3(4):403–6. PMID: 4607528.

[70] "Die „Droge Arzt“ und der Therapieerfolg." Springermedizin, 23 Nov. 2021, www.springermedizin.de/die-droge-arzt-und-der-therapieerfolg/16275800.

[71] Die „Droge Arzt" und der Therapieerfolg. Springermedizin, 3 May. 2021, www.springermedizin.de/die-droge-arzt-und-der-therapieerfolg/16275800.

[72] Colloca, Luana and Arthur J. Barsky. "Placebo and Nocebo Effects." N. Engl. J. Med., vol. 382, no. 6, 6 Feb. 2020, pp. 554–61. doi: https://doi.org/10.1056/NEJMra1907805.

1.11 Jesus Cleanses a Leper (Cleansing of a Leper)

1.11.1 Original Text (Luke 5:12–16; Mark 1:40–45; Matthew 8:1–4)

Jesus Cleanses a Leper (Luke 5:12–16): 12 While he was in one of the cities, there came a man full of leprosy. And when he saw Jesus, he fell on his face and begged him, "Lord, if you will, you can make me clean." 13 And Jesus stretched out his hand and touched him, saying, "I will; be clean." And immediately the leprosy left him. 14 And he charged him to tell no one, but "go and show yourself to the priest, and make an offering for your cleansing, as Moses commanded, for a proof to them." 15 But now even more the report about him went abroad, and great crowds gathered to hear him and to be healed of their infirmities. 16 But he would withdraw to desolate places and pray.

Jesus Cleanses a Leper (Mark 1:40–45): 40 And a leper came to him, imploring him, and kneeling said to him, "If you will, you can make me clean." 41 Moved with pity, he stretched out his hand and touched him and said to him, "I will; be clean." 42 And immediately the leprosy left him, and he was made clean. 43 And Jesus sternly charged him and sent him away at once, 44 and said to him, "See that you say nothing to anyone, but go, show yourself to the priest and offer for your cleansing what Moses commanded, for a proof to them." 45 But he went out and began to talk freely about it, and to spread the news, so that Jesus could no longer openly enter a town, but was out in desolate places, and people were coming to him from every quarter.

Jesus Cleanses a Leper (Matthew 8:1–4): 1 When he came down from the mountain, great crowds followed him. 2 And behold, a leper came to him and knelt before him, saying, "Lord, if you will, you can make me clean." 3 And Jesus stretched out his hand and touched him, saying, "I will; be clean." And immediately his leprosy was cleansed. 4 And Jesus said to him, "See that you say nothing to anyone, but go, show yourself to the priest and offer the gift that Moses commanded, for a proof to them."

1.11.2 Description and Interpretation

When a leprous man saw Jesus, he threw himself on his knees before him and said to Jesus, "Lord, if you are willing, you can make me clean." Jesus reached out his hand, touched him, and said, "I will - be made clean!" At the same moment, the man was freed from his leprosy. Jesus instructed the man not to tell anyone about this, but to show himself to a priest and offer a cleansing sacrifice.

When we hear this story of the "healing" of a leper, we always imagine that in Jesus' time, lepers were sick, disfigured cripples or people suffering from leprosy. Leprosy in Jesus' time did not mean a specific disease—the term disease did not even exist in Hebrew at that time—but rather **leprosy represented a *legal* status**: If someone was unclean, he had to live apart and stay outside the camp. Just as at the time of the pandemic (2019–2022) contact persons of people suffering from Covid-19 had to be quarantined and were forcibly segregated by notice and according to certain rules. What was done by the health authorities in our country was done by a rabbi at that time. An unclean person was thus leprous, segregated from others, i.e. socially isolated.

Who or what was to be considered "unclean" and what was to be done if the uncleanness was to be removed is described in detail in the 3rd Book of Moses (Leviticus 13:14). This included, for example, visible skin diseases, but also uncleanness and discolouration of clothes or houses. All these conditions led to the status of a leper. The "verdict" of pure or impure was pronounced by priests and was valid for a certain time, just as it is still done today by a quarantine notice. Nowadays, it is done by the health authority, but at that time it was done by a priest. Just as today an official can annul the decision, at that time a priest or rabbi could declare someone clean again. **Jesus lectured in the synagogues and was considered a rabbi, so he was able to rid someone of leprosy by touch**. Nowhere in this example is there any mention of *healing*, but only of "deliverance from leprosy", i.e. a kind of "acquittal", which by its very nature has an "instantaneous" effect.

Even though the Hebrew term "leprosy" (Zaraat) was repeatedly translated with the Greek term "lepros", this did not mean that the affected person suffered from leprosy. Rather, all people were segregated or considered unclean if they had any outward sign of uncleanness. This included all skin diseases that appeared suspect such as the perfectly harmless white spot disease (vitiligo), psoriasis and most forms of a skin rash (exanthema). To the extent that these skin diseases existed for a lifetime, the "status of uncleanness" was also often maintained for a lifetime (Leviticus 13:1–18, 13:1–59).[73] And just as today a health authority official in the COVID-19 pandemic did not dare to cancel a segregation order, even if it was completely nonsensical from a medical point of view, priests did not dare to classify lepers as clean again if all rules according to Leviticus 13:1–18[74] for the cancellation of leprosy were not fulfilled. Jesus was different here and overrode many a nonsensical rule, but instructed those affected to perform the prescribed sacrifices. Interesting detail on the side: apparently one recognized already at that time that clothes and objects could be infectious. Therefore, clothes and houses could also be considered unclean and then had to be avoided (Leviticus 14:44–55),[75] were "quarantined," so to speak.

The term "leper" is often equated with "leprosy", which is not quite correct. In the German language, the term leprosy appeared at the end of the eighteenth century and replaced terms such as "segregated". In Greek, the term lepros has

[73] *3.Mose 13,1–59, "Einheitsübersetzung 2016:: ERF Bibleserver." 23 Nov. 2021*, www.bibleserver.com/EU/3.Mose13%2C1-59.

[74] 3.Mose 14,1–57, "Einheitsübersetzung 2016:: ERF Bibleserver." 23 Nov. 2021, www.bibleserver.com/EU/3.Mose14.

[75] 3.Mose 14,44–55, "Einheitsübersetzung 2016:: ERF Bibleserver." 23 Nov. 2021, www.bibleserver.com/EU/3.Mose14.

been known since ancient times and meant "scaly" or "rough." The Hebrew term "Zaraat" as used in Leviticus 13 and 14 encompasses skin diseases and not leprosy.[76] However, in the Septuagint this term has been translated into Greek as lepros.[77] In today's translation of the Bible ("German Einheitsübersetzung") the word leprosy does not appear, while it is still present in English and Spanish translations.[78]

So, we can assume that in the Bible people were called lepers who, according to Leviticus 13, met the criteria mentioned above and about whom the population was afraid that the disease could be transmitted to healthy people, so to speak. At that time, people had no idea about infectious diseases. Nevertheless, people were afraid of the transmission of "uncleanliness", especially since there was already the observation at that time that certain changes occurred epidemically. This did not only apply to infectious diseases, but also to afflictions occurring throughout the country, for example poisoning with ergot, which led to the clinical picture of ergotism.[79]

At that time, the lepers must have been cared for by other people, otherwise they could not have survived. Apparently, Jesus noticed that the people who cared for the lepers did not necessarily fall ill themselves. So he could assume that the leprosy was actually mainly a social isolation and did not necessarily make them sick. They were simply socially isolated people, "outcasts" from society. People did not want to have anything to do with them, because they were afraid of them and did not know how to deal with them. Leviticus chapter 13 described exactly who is to be considered a leper and Leviticus chapter 14 described, when the leprosy was to be lifted again. As I said, this can best be compared with today's quarantine rules. One can imagine that life for a leper of that time was quite cruel. Probably many died from isolation alone. Likewise, one can well imagine that it bothered Jesus that some people experienced unnecessary social exclusion. It was therefore convenient for him if he could set examples to reintegrate these people socially by declaring them "pure".

Similar behaviour was seen in our country toward AIDS patients until a few years ago. At that time, when the disease was newly discovered and there were

---

76 Autoren der Wikimedia-Projekte. "Lepra – Wikipedia." 23 Oct. 2003, de.wikipedia.org/w/index.php?title=Lepra&oldid=217269184.

77 "Zur Heilung des Aussätzigen in Mk 1, 39–45 – Auslegungssache." 24 Nov. 2021, auslegungssache.at/5531/zur-heilung-des-aussaetzigen-in-mk-1-39-45.

78 ""lepra" | Einheitsübersetzung 2016:: ERF Bibleserver." 24 Nov. 2021, www.bibleserver.com/search/EU/lepra.

79 Bauer, Veit Harold. "Das Antonius-Feuer in Kunst und Medizin." Ergotismus-Epidemien in der Überlieferung vom Altertum bis heute. Springer, 1973, pp. 33–51. doi: https://doi.org/10.1007/978-3-642-65768-9_6.

no treatment options, they were also ostracized. Healthy people no longer dared to shake hands with these people for fear of catching the disease. They were also no longer invited by healthy people and no longer went out with them, so that these people were socially isolated, at least initially. In the current Covid-19 pandemic, collective "leprosy" is again taking place, so to speak, as the majority of the vaccinated try to exclude the unvaccinated.

The burden of leprosy was probably not only the actual disease, but above all the social exclusion. Isolation and lack of social support in itself leads to illness and shortened life expectancy.[80] The mere expulsion of a person from society leads to a number of ailments and diseases. Mental illnesses can also be mentioned here.[81] And here Jesus could probably show his strength. Social exclusion was unacceptable, especially for a person like Jesus, who preached charity and told stories like the Good Samaritan. Social exclusion went against his basic attitude. For this reason alone, he had to show the public that it was okay to have contact with lepers. Yes, that it is even good for the lepers if one deals with them and accepts them as they are. We know from modern studies that healing processes are initiated or accelerated by social support alone. Seen in this light, Jesus can be considered the first "social psychologist" or "social physician". Similar to the socialist and physician Viktor Adler in the nineteenth century, who experienced the excessive poverty of the Viennese brick workers and then intervened on their behalf. He alone freed them from their poverty and their "leprosy".

The "miracle healing" should therefore not be seen as the immediate disappearance of all external signs, but rather in the fact that Jesus showed that he was not afraid of these people. By reaching out his hand to a leper, that leper was instantly reintegrated socially and was no longer a leper. The leper described was only described as unclean without any external signs of disease.

[80] Pantel, Johannes. "Gesundheitliche Risiken von Einsamkeit und sozialer Isolation im Alter." Geriatr. Rep., vol. 16, no. 1, 1 Mar. 2021, pp. 6–8. doi: https://doi.org/10.1007/s42090-020-1225-0.

[81] Noor, Masi, et al. "The social psychology of collective victimhood." Eur. J. Soc. Psychol., vol. 47, no. 2, 1 Mar. 2017, pp. 121–34. doi: https://doi.org/10.1002/ejsp.2300.

Abstract: No miracle cure, but restoration of normal legal status (cancellation of a quarantine).

Laws About Leprosy (Leviticus 13:1–59): 1 The Lord spoke to Moses and Aaron, saying,
2 When a person has on the skin of his body a swelling or an eruption or a spot, and it turns into a case of leprous disease on the skin of his body, then he shall be brought to Aaron the priest or to one of his sons the priests,
3 and the priest shall examine the diseased area on the skin of his body. And if the hair in the diseased area has turned white and the disease appears to be deeper than the skin of his body, it is a case of leprous disease. When the priest has examined him, he shall pronounce him unclean.
4 But if the spot is white in the skin of his body and appears no deeper than the skin, and the hair in it has not turned white, the priest shall shut up the diseased person for seven days.
5 And the priest shall examine him on the seventh day, and if in his eyes the disease is checked and the disease has not spread in the skin, then the priest shall shut him up for another seven days.
6 And the priest shall examine him again on the seventh day, and if the diseased area has faded and the disease has not spread in the skin, then the priest shall pronounce him clean; it is only an eruption. And he shall wash his clothes and be clean.
7 But if the eruption spreads in the skin, after he has shown himself to the priest for his cleansing, he shall appear again before the priest.
8 And the priest shall look, and if the eruption has spread in the skin, then the priest shall pronounce him unclean; it is a leprous disease.
9 When a man is afflicted with a leprous disease, he shall be brought to the priest,
10 and the priest shall look. And if there is a white swelling in the skin that has turned the hair white, and there is raw flesh in the swelling,
11 it is a chronic leprous disease in the skin of his body, and the priest shall pronounce him unclean. He shall not shut him up, for he is unclean.
12 And if the leprous disease breaks out in the skin, so that the leprous disease covers all the skin of the diseased person from head to foot, so far as the priest can see,
13 then the priest shall look, and if the leprous disease has covered all his body, he shall pronounce him clean of the disease; it has all turned white, and he is clean.
14 But when raw flesh appears on him, he shall be unclean.
15 And the priest shall examine the raw flesh and pronounce him unclean. Raw flesh is unclean, for it is a leprous disease.
16 But if the raw flesh recovers and turns white again, then he shall come to the priest,
17 and the priest shall examine him, and if the disease has turned white, then the priest shall pronounce the diseased person clean; he is clean.
18 "If there is in the skin of one's body a boil and it heals,
19 and in the place of the boil there comes a white swelling or a reddish-white spot, then it shall be shown to the priest.
20 And the priest shall look, and if it appears deeper than the skin and its hair has turned white, then the priest shall pronounce him unclean. It is a case of leprous disease that has broken out in the boil.
21 But if the priest examines it, and there is no white hair in it and it is not deeper than the skin, but has faded, then the priest shall shut him up seven days.
22 And if it spreads in the skin, then the priest shall pronounce him unclean; it is a disease.
23 But if the spot remains in one place and does not spread, it is the scar of the boil, and the priest shall pronounce him clean.
24 "Or, when the body has a burn on its skin and the raw flesh of the burn becomes a spot, reddish-white or white,
25 the priest shall examine it, and if the hair in the spot has turned white, and it appears deeper than the skin, then it is a leprous disease. It has broken out in the burn, and the priest shall pronounce him unclean; it is a case of leprous disease.
26 But if the priest examines it and there is no white hair in the spot, and it is no deeper than the skin, but has faded, the priest shall shut him up seven days,
27 and the priest shall examine him the seventh day. If it is spreading in the skin, then the priest shall pronounce him unclean; it is a case of leprous disease.
28 But if the spot remains in one place and does not spread in the skin, but has faded, it is a swelling from the burn, and the priest shall pronounce him clean, for it is the scar of the burn.
29 When a man or woman has a disease on the head or the beard,
30 the priest shall examine the disease. And if it appears deeper than the skin, and the hair in it is yellow and thin, then the priest shall pronounce him unclean. It is an itch, a leprous disease of the head or the beard.
31 And if the priest examines the itching disease, and it appears no deeper than the skin and

there is no black hair in it, then the priest shall shut up the person with the itching disease for seven days, 32 and on the seventh day the priest shall examine the disease. If the itch has not spread, and there is in it no yellow hair, and the itch appears to be no deeper than the skin, 33 then he shall shave himself, but the itch he shall not shave; and the priest shall shut up the person with the itching disease for another seven days. 34 And on the seventh day the priest shall examine the itch, and if the itch has not spread in the skin, and it appears to be no deeper than the skin, then the priest shall pronounce him clean. And he shall wash his clothes and be clean. 35 But if the itch spreads in the skin after his cleansing, 36 then the priest shall examine him, and if the itch has spread in the skin, the priest need not seek for the yellow hair; he is unclean. 37 But if in his eyes the itch is unchanged and black hair has grown in it, the itch is healed and he is clean, and the priest shall pronounce him clean. 38 When a man or a woman has spots on the skin of the body, white spots, 39 the priest shall look, and if the spots on the skin of the body are of a dull white, it is leucoderma that has broken out in the skin; he is clean. 40 If a man's hair falls out from his head, he is bald; he is clean. 41 And if a man's hair falls out from his forehead, he has baldness of the forehead; he is clean. 42 But if there is on the bald head or the bald forehead a reddish-white diseased area, it is a leprous disease breaking out on his bald head or his bald forehead. 43 Then the priest shall examine him, and if the diseased swelling is reddish-white on his bald head or on his bald forehead, like the appearance of leprous disease in the skin of the body, 44 he is a leprous man, he is unclean. The priest must pronounce him unclean; his disease is on his head. 45 The leprous person who has the disease shall wear torn clothes and let the hair of his head hang loose, and he shall cover his upper lip and cry out, 'Unclean, unclean.' 46 He shall remain unclean as long as he has the disease. He is unclean. He shall live alone. His dwelling shall be outside the camp. 47 When there is a case of leprous disease in a garment, whether a woollen or a linen garment, 48 in warp or woof of linen or wool, or in a skin or in anything made of skin, 49 if the disease is greenish or reddish in the garment, or in the skin or in the warp or the woof or in any article made of skin, it is a case of leprous disease, and it shall be shown to the priest. 50 And the priest shall examine the disease and shut up that which has the disease for seven days. 51 Then he shall examine the disease on the seventh day. If the disease has spread in the garment, in the warp or the woof, or in the skin, whatever be the use of the skin, the disease is a persistent leprous disease; it is unclean. 52 And he shall burn the garment, or the warp or the woof, the wool or the linen, or any article made of skin that is diseased, for it is a persistent leprous disease. It shall be burned in the fire. 53 And if the priest examines, and if the disease has not spread in the garment, in the warp or the woof or in any article made of skin, 54 then the priest shall command that they wash the thing in which is the disease, and he shall shut it up for another seven days. 55 And the priest shall examine the diseased thing after it has been washed. And if the appearance of the diseased area has not changed, though the disease has not spread, it is unclean. You shall burn it in the fire, whether the rot is on the back or on the front. 56 But if the priest examines, and if the diseased area has faded after it has been washed, he shall tear it out of the garment or the skin or the warp or the woof. 57 Then if it appears again in the garment, in the warp or the woof, or in any article made of skin, it is spreading. You shall burn with fire whatever has the disease. 58 But the garment, or the warp or the woof, or any article made of skin from which the disease departs when you have washed it, shall then be washed a second time, and be clean. 59 This is the law for a case of leprous disease in a garment of wool or linen, either in the warp or the woof, or in any article made of skin, to determine whether it is clean or unclean.

1.12 Jesus Heals a Paralytic (Healing of the Paralytic After Forgiveness of Sins)

1.12.1 Original Text of the Bible (Luke 5:17–26; Mark 2:1–12, Matthew 9:1–8)

Jesus Heals a Paralytic (Luke 5:17–26): 17 On one of those days, as he was teaching, Pharisees and teachers of the law were sitting there, who had come from every village of Galilee and Judea and from Jerusalem. And the power of the Lord was with him to heal. 18 And behold, some men were bringing on a bed a man who was paralysed, and they were seeking to bring him in and lay him before Jesus, 19 but finding no way to bring him in, because of the crowd, they went up on the roof and let him down with his bed through the tiles into the midst before Jesus. 20 And when he saw their faith, he said, "Man, your sins are forgiven you." 21 And the scribes and the Pharisees began to question, saying, "Who is this who speaks blasphemies? Who can forgive sins but God alone?" 22 When Jesus perceived their thoughts, he answered them, "Why do you question in your hearts? 23 Which is easier, to say, 'Your sins are forgiven you,' or to say, 'Rise and walk'? 24 But that you may know that the Son of Man has authority on earth to forgive sins"—he said to the man who was paralysed—"I say to you, rise, pick up your bed and go home." 25 And immediately he rose up before them and picked up what he had been lying on and went home, glorifying God. 26 And amazement seized them all, and they glorified God and were filled with awe, saying, "We have seen extraordinary things today."

Jesus Heals a Paralytic (Mark 2:1–12): 1 And when he returned to Capernaum after some days, it was reported that he was at home. 2 And many were gathered together, so that there was no more room, not even at the door. And he was preaching the word to them. 3 And they came, bringing to him a paralytic carried by four men. 4 And when they could not get near him because of the crowd, they removed the roof above him, and when they had made an opening, they let down the bed on which the paralytic lay. 5 And when Jesus saw their faith, he said to the paralytic, "Son, your sins are forgiven." 6 Now some of the scribes were sitting there, questioning in their hearts, 7 "Why does this man speak like that? He is blaspheming! Who can forgive sins but God alone?" 8 And immediately Jesus, perceiving in his spirit that they thus questioned within themselves, said to them, "Why do you question these things in your hearts? 9 Which is easier, to say to the paralytic, 'Your sins are forgiven,' or to say, 'Rise, take up your bed and walk'? 10 But that you may know that the Son of Man has authority on earth to forgive sins"—he said to the paralytic— 11 "I say to you, rise, pick up your bed, and go home." 12 And he rose and immediately picked up his bed and went out before them all, so that they were all amazed and glorified God, saying, "We never saw anything like this!".

Jesus Heals a Paralytic (Matthew 9:1–8): 1 And getting into a boat, he crossed over and came to his own city. 2 And behold, some people brought to him a paralytic, lying on a bed. And when Jesus saw their faith, he said to the paralytic, "Take heart, my son; your sins are forgiven." 3 And behold, some of the scribes said to themselves, "This man is blaspheming." 4 But Jesus, knowing their thoughts, said, "Why do you think evil in your hearts? 5 For which is easier, to say, 'Your sins are forgiven,' or to say, 'Rise and walk'? 6 But that you may know that the Son of Man has authority on earth to forgive sins"—he then said to the paralytic—"Rise, pick up your bed and go home." 7 And he rose and went home. 8 When the crowds saw it, they were afraid, and they glorified God, who had given such authority to men.

1.12.2 Description and Interpretation

There was a large crowd in front of the house where Jesus was staying. Some men wanted to bring a paralytic to Jesus, but could not get through the crowd. They decided to go up on the roof, remove some roof tiles there, so that they could lower the paralytic inside the house. Jesus was amazed at the strong faith in him that these men had and said to the paralytic, "Your sins are forgiven". This angered the scribes who were there, as they felt it was blasphemy for Jesus to forgive sins. Only God could forgive sins. Jesus noticed this anger and said to them "so that you may know that I can forgive sins, look here everyone". He turned to the paralytic and told him to get up and go home. To everyone's amazement, the paralytic got up, took his camp bed and went home.

In this case, a man who apparently could not move is brought to Jesus. Whether he had been paralysed for years or only for a few minutes or hours is not clear from the Bible. In any case, the man in question could be healed with a **suggestive command "get up, take your bed and go home". This points to a psychogenic paralysis**. Psychogenic paralysis is not that uncommon in children,[82] and gets little attention in the medical world.[83] If you enter the search term "psychogenic paralysis" in Google, you get 33,800 hits and in the medical database PubMed there are 151 articles on this topic.[84]

The diagnosis of "psychogenic paralysis" does not even take into account the paralysis symptoms that can occur in the context of **hyperventilation tetany in anxiety disorders** or in the context of a panic attack. Anyone who has experienced a person with acute hyperventilation (breathing too fast and too deep) in the context of a panic attack knows how "dangerous" the situation can look. Every doctor who has already treated such diseases knows how quickly one can feel like a "miracle worker" here. As a rule, in such an "emergency situation" today, one will administer to such patients a sedating drug in the form of an intravenous injection. Sometimes, however, the mere presence of the doctor and the prospect of a cure is enough for a patient to experience a "miracle cure". Thus, it happens again and again that a doctor is called to patients who have a panic attack with symptoms of paralysis. For the doctor, this form of paralysis is a visual diagnosis, because the affected people show so-called **carpopedal spasms**. For the layman, the term "paw position" of the hands is more descriptive. In the full-blown case, however, there is not only paralysis in the hands (with paw position), but also paralysis of the feet, which leads to immobility. In this form of paralysis, the following happens: the affected person, who for some

---

[82] Nowak M. Psychogene Lähmungen im Kindes- und Jugendalter [Psychogenic paralysis in childhood and adolescence]. Z Kinder Jugendpsychiatr Psychother. 2002 Aug;30(3):199–210. German. doi: https://doi.org/10.1024//1422-4917.30.3.199. PMID: 12227222.

[83] Nowak DA, Fink GR. Psychogenic movement disorders: aetiology, phenomenology, neuroanatomical correlates and therapeutic approaches. Neuroimage. 2009 Sep;47(3):1015–25. doi: https://doi.org/10.1016/j.neuroimage.2009.04.082. Epub 2009 May 6. PMID: 19426818.

[84] "psychogenic paralysis - Search Results - PubMed." PubMed, 24 Nov. 2021, pubmed.ncbi.nlm.nih.gov/?term=psychogenic%20paralysis%20&page=2.

reason has become afraid (perhaps because he has just "sinned"), panics. The fear causes him to start breathing more deeply.

Deep breathing causes the body to lose too much CO_2, with the result that the pH of the blood rises. In medicine, this condition is called hyperventilation alkalosis. The alkalinization of the blood in turn results in an increase in the ability of calcium to bind to the proteins in the blood. Calcium is increasingly bound and is thus no longer available to the nerves in sufficient quantities for the transmission of nerve impulses. This disturbed transmission of nerve impulses is experienced by patients as very unpleasant: There is tingling in the hands and feet and circulatory disturbances (cold hands and feet) sometimes also in the face around the mouth area (perioral pallor). As a rule, these sensory disturbances lead to even more anxiety, which in turn leads to breathing not only deeper but also even faster. A vicious circle occurs: anxiety leads to hyperventilation with sensory disturbances, these lead to increased anxiety and further intensification of hyperventilation. In the full picture, something like this looks quite dramatic, eventually leading to paralysis in the face, hands, and feet (carpopedal spasms) and can even lead to unconsciousness. The medical profession refers to the paralysis symptoms caused in this way as hyperventilation tetany or hyperventilation syndrome.[85] If unconsciousness occurs, the body would then heal itself, because in unconsciousness the anxiety fades, breathing returns to normal and the patient "wakes up healthy again". Today, of course, doctors don't let it get that far and don't let the patient suffer for so long, but give a "sedative injection" straight away. While the nurse is preparing the sedative injection, the experienced and thus safe doctor will hold the patient's hand and convey calm. This measure alone, or the certainty that he or she is now being helped, can restore complete freedom from symptoms within a few seconds. Often the administration of the sedative injection is no longer even necessary, because just by "laying on of hands" or better by the calming of the external circumstances a "miracle healing" is accomplished. For relatives who have never experienced such conditions, this may indeed have represented a "miracle", although it was not one.

Jesus may have immediately recognized the fear in the eyes of the paralytic and "forgave his sins". By this alone he created an "authoritarian situation", so authoritarian that the scribes, who actually always claimed the authority for themselves, were annoyed and loudly upset about it. Jesus now had to "show them" and obviously spoke in command form "get up, take your bed and walk" (the best he could do at that moment from a therapeutic point of view) and lo and behold, normality suddenly returned to the "paralysed man". He could move normally again and actually get up and take his stretcher with him. Nice therapy success, but no miracle!

Emergency physicians regularly experience such situations, although it must be said that nowadays the situation described above is almost never seen in its full form even by emergency physicians. As a rule, the relatives, or surrounding people call

---

[85] Du Pasquier D, Fellrath JM, Sauty A. Syndrome d'hyperventilation et respiration dysfonctionnelle : mise à jour [Hyperventilation syndrome and dysfunctional breathing : update]. Rev Med Suisse. 2020 Jun 17;16(698):1243–1249. French. PMID: 32558453.

the ambulance so early that it almost never comes to the full picture of hyperventilation tetany. In the past, when Tyrolean mountain farmers called the ambulance relatively late in such cases, and when there was no emergency doctor to provide initial treatment on the spot, it took quite a long time for the affected person to get into the hands of the doctor. In addition, there were long transport routes. In those days, doctors could still see the full picture of hyperventilation and dramatic panic attacks were not at all uncommon.

But there is not only acute hyperventilation tetany with a dramatic course. Even among doctors, it is little known that there are also **"chronic" hyperventilation** and **chronic hyperventilation syndrome**. Young women in particular are affected when they begin to hyperventilate around ovulation due to hormones. This often lasts for days and leads to cold hands and feet and pallor. Parents then frequently call the affected girls a "pale creature".

Abstract: Psychogenic paralysis or psychogenic dystonia (ICD-10 F44.4) or paralysis in the context of (chronic) hyperventilation tetany (ICD-10 R06.4).

1.13 A Man with a Withered Hand (Healing of the Man with the Withered Hand on the Sabbath)

1.13.1 Original Text of the Bible (Luke 6:6–10; Mark 3:1–6; Matthew 12:9–14)

A Man with a Withered Hand (Luke 6:6–10): 6 On another Sabbath, he entered the synagogue and was teaching, and a man was there whose right hand was withered. 7 And the scribes and the Pharisees watched him, to see whether he would heal on the Sabbath, so that they might find a reason to accuse him. 8 But he knew their thoughts, and he said to the man with the withered hand, "Come and stand here." And he rose and stood there. 9 And Jesus said to them, "I ask you, is it lawful on the Sabbath to do good or to do harm, to save life or to destroy it?" 10 And after looking around at them all he said to him, "Stretch out your hand." And he did so, and his hand was restored. 11 But they were filled with fury and discussed with one another what they might do to Jesus.

A Man with a Withered Hand (Mark 3:1–6): 1 Again he entered the synagogue, and a man was there with a withered hand. 2 And they watched Jesus, to see whether he would heal him on the Sabbath, so that they might accuse him. 3 And he said to the man with the withered hand, "Come here." 4 And he said to them, "Is it lawful on the Sabbath to do good or to do harm, to save life or to kill?" But they were silent. 5 And he looked around at them with anger, grieved at their hardness of heart, and said to the man, "Stretch out your hand." He stretched it out, and his hand was restored. 6 The Pharisees went out and immediately held counsel with the Herodians against him, how to destroy him.

A Man with a Withered Hand (Matthew 12:9–14): 9 He went on from there and entered their synagogue. 10 And a man was there with a withered hand. And they asked him, "Is it lawful to heal on the Sabbath?"-so that they might accuse him. 11 He said to them, "Which one of you who has a sheep, if it falls into a pit on the Sabbath, will not take hold of it and lift it out? 12 Of how much more value is a man than a sheep! So it is lawful to do good on the Sabbath." 13 Then he said to the man, "Stretch out your hand." And the man stretched it out, and it was restored, healthy like the other. 14 But the Pharisees went out and conspired against him, how to destroy him.

1.13.2 Description and Interpretation

Jesus went to teach in the synagogue on a Sabbath. There was a man there who had a "withered hand". But on Sabbath it was forbidden to treat or heal anyone. Nevertheless, Jesus said to the man with the withered hand, "Stand up and stand here in our midst." He asked the audience in the round, "is it forbidden to do good or to save a life on the Sabbath?" After no one answered, he ordered the man to stretch out his hand. Immediately, the man's hand was healed. The Pharisees were apparently so annoyed by the healing success that they subsequently decided to kill Jesus.

Vasospasms (spasms of the vessels) often lead to impressive changes in the colour of the skin.[86] The fingers are mostly affected. If such vasospasms result in a "demarcation line", a line from which the fingers are white while the rest of the hand is still well supplied with blood, physicians refer to this condition as "Raynaud's phenomenon".[87] Vasospasms can be triggered by cold, stress, mental strain, carrying objects or manual work.[88] If regular "attacks" with visible circulatory disturbance occur, the condition is referred to as Raynaud's disease.[89] The disease is named after the French physician Maurice Raynaud (1834–1881). In the past, it was also called "**Digitus mortuus (dead man's finger)**"[90] because the fingers or hand could be as pale as those of a dead person.

This phenomenon is also not so rare. If one also includes mild preliminary stages of this circulatory disorder, it occurs in up to 20% of construction workers, up to 40% of forestry workers, and up to 50% of ore miners. Approximately 5–10% of the population is thought to have developed Raynaud's syndrome at some time during their lives.[91] A familial clustering is also found. The Raynaud's phenomenon is also frequently observed in women who are not manually active, and it occurs here not

[86] Takáts A, Garai I, Papp G, Hevér T, Csiki E, András C, Csiki Z. Raynaud-szindróma, 2011 [Raynaud's syndrome, 2011]. Orv Hetil. 2012 Mar 18;153(11):403–9. Hungarian. doi: https://doi.org/10.1556/OH.2012.29321. PMID: 22390864.

[87] Gary T., Brodmann M. Raynaudphänomen: Raynaudphänomen. Ärztewoche; RheumaPlus 2007: pp. 17–20.

[88] Weigel I, Klein-Weigel P, Kinzl J, Biebl W, Fraedrich G, Heidrich H. Psychometrische Tests bei primärem Raynaud-Phänomen--Untersuchungsergebnisse an einem Tiroler Patientenkollektiv [Psychometric investigation of Tyrolean patients with primary Raynaud's phenomenon]. Wien Med Wochenschr. 2006 Nov;156(21–22):574–82. German. doi: https://doi.org/10.1007/s10354-006-0338-x. PMID: 17160374.

[89] Temprano KK. A Review of Raynaud's Disease. Mo Med. 2016 Mar–Apr;113(2):123–6. PMID: 27311222; PMCID: PMC6139949.

[90] Lemmens, H. A. J. "Raynaud-Phänomen—Angina manus et digitorum—Digitus mortuus." Acta Chir. Austriaca, vol. 9, no. 5, 1 Sept. 1977, pp. 134–5. doi: https://doi.org/10.1007/BF02601013.

[91] Gary T., Brodmann M. Raynaudphänomen: Raynaudphänomen. Ärztewoche; RheumaPlus 2007: pp. 17–20.

only in the cold, but above all also under psychological stress.[92] Doctors who deal with Raynaud's disease also like to treat this disease in the symptom-free interval with psychotropic drugs (so-called SSRI) which are actually approved for the treatment of depression and for the treatment of anxiety. **Anxiety and cold hands are well-known triggers**[93] and, as mentioned above, have a lot to do with each other, as hyperventilation also plays a certain role here. We have seen above that **hyperventilation leads to disturbances in nerve transmission and thus to disturbances in vascular regulation**. This regulation disturbance leads in the **minimum case only to cold hands (normal reaction), in the maximum variant to the Raynaud phenomenon or "dead finger"**. Anxiety can therefore be regarded as a trigger for a Raynaud's attack. However, the cause of this disorder is more complex and not always ascertainable. The causes of Raynaud's disease range from autoimmune diseases to the occurrence of vasospasms in the context of a paraneoplastic syndrome associated with cancer. As mentioned, the triggers—but not the cause—are often psychological. Thus, Raynaud's phenomenon may disappear as quickly as it occurred. In this case, Jesus' instant success may have been due to the relief of anxiety.

Alternatively, the withered hand could have been CRPS (complex regional pain syndrome, formerly called algodystrophy or Sudeck disease). In this case, physical trauma, psychological trauma, thrombosis, or rheumatic diseases may be possible triggers.[94] Complex regional pain syndrome is also a neurovegetative condition.

Abstract: Raynaud's disease (ICD-10 I73.0) or CRPS (complex regional pain syndrome, ICD-10 M89.0).

---

[92] Weigel I, Klein-Weigel P, Kinzl J, Biebl W, Fraedrich G, Heidrich H. Psychometrische Tests bei primärem Raynaud-Phänomen--Untersuchungsergebnisse an einem Tiroler Patientenkollektiv [Psychometric investigation of Tyrolean patients with primary Raynaud's phenomenon]. Wien Med Wochenschr. 2006 Nov;156(21–22):574–82. German. doi: https://doi.org/10.1007/s10354-006-0338-x. PMID: 17160374.

[93] Brown KM, Middaugh SJ, Haythornthwaite JA, Bielory L. The effects of stress, anxiety, and outdoor temperature on the frequency and severity of Raynaud's attacks: the Raynaud's Treatment Study. J Behav Med. 2001 Apr;24(2):137–53. doi: https://doi.org/10.1023/a:1010758530555. PMID: 11392916.

[94] Deutscher Ärzteverlag GmbH, Redaktion. "Morbus Sudeck: Bezeichnung unpassend." Deutsches Ärzteblatt, 23 Feb. 2018, www.aerzteblatt.de/archiv/196452/Morbus-Sudeck-Bezeichnung-unpassend.

1.14 Jesus Heals a Centurion's Servant (The Distant Healing of the Servant of a Roman Officer in Capernaum)

1.14.1 Original Text of the Bible (Luke 7:1–10; Matthew 8:5–13)

Jesus Heals a Centurion's Servant (Luke 7:1–10): 1 After he had finished all his sayings in the hearing of the people, he entered Capernaum. 2 Now a centurion had a servant who was sick and at the point of death, who was highly valued by him. 3 When the centurion heard about Jesus, he sent to him elders of the Jews, asking him to come and heal his servant. 4 And when they came to Jesus, they pleaded with him earnestly, saying, "He is worthy to have you do this for him, 5 for he loves our nation, and he is the one who built us our synagogue." 6 And Jesus went with them. When he was not far from the house, the centurion sent friends, saying to him, "Lord, do not trouble yourself, for I am not worthy to have you come under my roof. 7 Therefore I did not presume to come to you. But say the word, and let my servant be healed. 8 For I too am a man set under authority, with soldiers under me: and I say to one, 'Go,' and he goes; and to another, 'Come,' and he comes; and to my servant, 'Do this,' and he does it." 9 When Jesus heard these things, he marveled at him, and turning to the crowd that followed him, said, "I tell you, not even in Israel have I found such faith." 10 And when those who had been sent returned to the house, they found the servant well.

The Faith of a Centurion (Matthew 8:5–13): 5 When he had entered Capernaum, a centurion came forward to him, appealing to him, 6 "Lord, my servant is lying paralyzed at home, suffering terribly." 7 And he said to him, "I will come and heal him." 8 But the centurion replied, "Lord, I am not worthy to have you come under my roof, but only say the word, and my servant will be healed. 9 For I too am a man under authority, with soldiers under me. And I say to one, 'Go,' and he goes, and to another, 'Come,' and he comes, and to my servant, 'Do this,' and he does it." 10 When Jesus heard this, he marveled and said to those who followed him, "Truly, I tell you, with no one in Israel have I found such faith. 11 I tell you, many will come from east and west and recline at table with Abraham, Isaac, and Jacob in the kingdom of heaven, 12 while the sons of the kingdom will be thrown into the outer darkness. In that place there will be weeping and gnashing of teeth." 13 And to the centurion Jesus said, "Go; let it be done for you as you have believed." And the servant was healed at that very moment.

1.14.2 Description and Interpretation

A captain had a servant whom he valued very much and who was lying at home paralyzed and in great pain. He was afraid that his servant might die. When the centurion heard about Jesus, he asked Jesus to heal his servant. Jesus answered him that he was ready to come to his house and heal his servant. But the centurion said to Jesus, "he is not worthy for such a holy man as Jesus to come into his house. He should only give the order for his servant to be healed, and that would be enough to bring about a cure." Jesus was amazed at how much the centurion believed in him and his abilities. He said, "I have never found such faith in anyone. Therefore, it shall be done as you have believed". That same hour, the centurion found that his servant was healed.

Medically, this story in Luke's Gospel does not reveal much, especially since there is no description of what ailment the Roman soldier's servant was suffering from. In the Gospel of Matthew, only pain and symptoms of paralysis are mentioned. This suggests at first a **peripheral paralysis**, of a nerve that is "pinched" or a so-called **nerve compression syndrome**. Centrally caused paralysis does not cause pain, so this cause can be largely ruled out. Peripheral paralysis, whether due to a herniated disc or nerve compression syndrome, **is usually accompanied by increased muscle tension**. The problem with these conditions is that the pain leads to increased muscle tension, and the increased muscle tension in turn leads to increased pain,[95]a vicious circle that today would be treated with a muscle relaxant or a sedative injection in addition to painkillers. However, there are also supposed "miracle healers" today who can exert such a pronounced psychological effect on patients that they can eliminate pain simply by appearing or laying hands on them. We know that the knowledge that help is in sight, already cures a lot.[96] Psychologists would speak here also of "self-fulfilling prophecy". Physicians speak of the placebo effect. Probably, the servant was influenced by his master's strong belief in Jesus' healing powers. Thus, his medical condition improved at once when he heard that such a 'miraculous' intervention was likely to be applied to him.

Jesus already recognized at that time how important faith in something is.[97] Success occurs only if one also believes in it. If even a Roman (!), a member of the unbelievers, not to say of the heretical occupying power, suddenly believes in Jesus, then Jesus could be sure that this person could be strongly influenced by him. So he could say with good feeling "Go home quietly, your faith has helped you" and trust that his prophecy would be fulfilled by itself.[98]

The miracle lies rather in the fact that Jesus already 2000 years ago used suggestive methods[99] and understood how to use fundamental psychological processes in humans, which we all share to some extent. Perhaps the servant of the Roman officer was lying down with back pain and therefore could hardly move and could not work. When you see how often good physiotherapists achieve immediate pain relief just by touching the "right spot", you can see how effective such placebo effects are. It

[95] Hoffmann, S. O. and U. T. Egle. "Psychologische Schmerztherapie." Psychodynamische Konzepte bei somatoformen Schmerzzuständen. Springer, 2004, pp. 119-35. doi: https://doi.org/10.1007/978-3-662-09587-4_6.

[96] Balint, Enid. "Michael Balint und die Droge "Arzt"." Psyche, vol. 30, no. 2, 1976, pp. 105–24, https://elibrary.klett-cotta.de/article/99.120105/ps-30-2-105.

[97] Biser, Eugen. "Kann Glaube heilen?: Zur Frage nach Sinn und Wesen einer therapeutischen Theologie." Archive for the Psychology of Religion, vol. 21, no. 1, 1 Jan. 1994, pp. 19–36. doi: https://doi.org/10.1163/157361294X00039.

[98] Glaser, Christian. "Risiko im Management: 100 Fehler, Irrtümer, Verzerrungen und wie man sie vermeidet." Selbsterfüllende Prophezeiung. Springer Gabler, 7 May. 2019, pp. 81–84. doi: https://doi.org/10.1007/978-3-658-25835-1_21.

[99] Stokvis, Berthold and Manfred Pflanz. "Suggestion in der Medizin." Dtsch. Med. Wochenschr., vol. 86, no. 06, Feb. 1961, pp. 237–43. doi: https://doi.org/10.1055/s-0028-1112775.

usually doesn't matter at all which point the physical therapist touches, massages or presses, the only important thing is that the physical therapist believes in it and that the patient believes in it. The same applies to acupuncture, although here this phenomenon has already been studied and confirmed.[100]

The remarkable thing about this narration is that a Roman, who still believed in "primitive" polytheism, trusted Jesus more than his Jewish followers did. The Jews, who were from the "chosen" people, were supposed to believe in him (Jesus). Jesus reproached his followers for this and even "threatened" them that if they continued to be of little faith, the Romans would be more likely to "sit at table" with Abraham in the afterlife than the members of his own people.

Jesus knew about the power of faith and the power of suggestion. So he gave the Roman centurion the command he wanted, with which he was satisfied. The Bible records only that the servant experienced a spontaneous healing in the meantime. How and what happened in the meantime is not reported in the Bible.

"**Remote healing**" is apparently a widespread wishful thinking of many people, even today. If you enter the search term "remote healing" in Google, it gives 50.6 million (!) hits. Remote suggestion and remote hypnosis seem to profit from telecommunication and the internet and spread all over the world. A whole branch of industry apparently makes millions in sales with it, or with the belief in healing and the placebo effect associated with it. Placebo effects and self-fulfilling prophecies are not miracles, but the "normal" consequence of strong faith. Remote healing therefore "works" better with believers[101] than with non-believers.[102] The power of faith and suggestion is described by Jesus again and again, for example when he talks about faith that can move mountains. Finally, if you enter the search term "remote healing" in the scientific medical database PubMed, you will still find 926 hits (2022) for this keyword.

Abstract: Spinal pain syndrome with paralysis (ICD-10 M54) coded differently depending on location, e.g. low back pain syndrome (ICD-10 M54.5) or nerve compression syndrome (ICD-10 G58). Here, too, the coding depends on the localization, e.g., meralgia paraesthetica (inguinal tunnel syndrome) (ICD-10 G57.1).

---

[100] E. Ernst: Acupuncture—a critical analysis. In: Journal of Internal Medicine. 259, Nr. 2, 2006, S. 125–137. doi: https://doi.org/10.1111/j.1365-2796.2005.01584.x. PMID 16420542.

[101] Masters, Kevin S. "Research on the Healing Power of Distant Intercessory Prayer: Disconnect between Science and Faith." Journal of Psychology and Theology, vol. 33, no. 4, 1 Dec. 2005, pp. 268–77. doi: https://doi.org/10.1177/009164710503300403.

[102] Aviles JM, Whelan SE, Hernke DA, Williams BA, Kenny KE, O'Fallon WM, Kopecky SL. Intercessory prayer and cardiovascular disease progression in a coronary care unit population: a randomized controlled trial. Mayo Clin Proc. 2001 Dec;76(12):1192–8. doi: https://doi.org/10.4065/76.12.1192. PMID: 11761499.

1.15 Jesus Raises a Widow's Son (The Awakening of the Young Man of Naïn)

1.15.1 Original Text (Luke 7:11–17)

Jesus Raises a Widow's Son (Luke 7:11–17): 11 Soon afterward he went to a town called Naïn, and his disciples and a great crowd went with him. 12 As he drew near to the gate of the town, behold, a man who had died was being carried out, the only son of his mother, and she was a widow, and a considerable crowd from the town was with her. 13 And when the Lord saw her, he had compassion on her and said to her, "Do not weep." 14 Then he came up and touched the bier, and the bearers stood still. And he said, "Young man, I say to you, arise." 15 And the dead man sat up and began to speak, and Jesus gave him to his mother. 16 Fear seized them all, and they glorified God, saying, "A great prophet has arisen among us!" and "God has visited his people!" 17 And this report about him spread through the whole of Judea and all the surrounding country.

1.15.2 Description and Interpretation

Jesus entered the city of Naïn, followed by a large crowd. When he arrived there at the city gate, the people carried the deceased son of a widow out of the city on a bier. Many people accompanied the funeral procession. When Jesus saw the mother who had lost her only son, he had compassion on her and said to her, "do not weep." He approached the bier so that the bearers of the bier stopped and said to the deceased: "Young man, I tell you, get up!". Then the dead man sat up and began to speak. Jesus thus gave the son back to his mother.

At first sight, everything looks like a raising of the dead. However, the description suggests a classical case of "**apparent death**".[103] As described in the chapter "Determination of Death", the determination of certain death is really not easy. Mistakes in the determination of death were made again and again and still occur today, despite the assistance of technical devices.

In most cultures, there are terms like "apparent death". In Latin, such a state is also called "Vita Minima". Not only is there a loss of consciousness, but also the pulse and breathing become so weak that they can no longer be perceived by others. In the German area, the term "Scheintod" was used for the first time by the physician Dr. J. G. Krünitz in 1788.[104] Before that, people were apparently not even aware that there could be a state similar to death, but in which death had not actually occurred.

[103] Brandt L, Artmeier-Brandt U: Vom Scheintod zur Notfallmedizin. Wie eine als irrational erscheinende Furcht die Entstehung einer rationalen Medizin katalysierte. Anästh Intensivmed 2016;57:274–288 Aktiv Druck & Verlag Gmb; https://www.ai-online.info/images/ai-ausgabe/2016/05-2016/2016_5_274-288_Vom%20Scheintod%20zur%20Notfallmedizin.pdf.

[104] Autoren der Wikimedia-Projekte. "Scheintod – Wikipedia." 14 Sept. 2004, de.wikipedia.org/w/index.php?title=Scheintod&oldid=217070636.

In ancient times, it was common to "call the dead person by name several times to establish death if he did not answer".[105] A rather uncertain way to establish death.

Probably in the past, many people were buried alive because of lack of knowledge whether death had certainly occurred. Apparently, this was also suspected in the past. Especially in the Age of Enlightenment from the seventeenth century to the nineteenth century, there was great fear in Europe of being buried alive.[106] Therefore, people were given a "death bell" in the coffin. With it, the dead should be able to make themselves noticeable, if they were still alive. The laying out of the dead may also have been justified by this, because people's fears of being buried alive always accompanied them.

In the Mediterranean countries it was, and still is, customary to bury a dead person very quickly. Thus, even today in some countries, dead bodies must be buried within 24 h. It may be assumed that in this period of time relatively many people who were unconscious for some reason were buried alive. This was probably the case with the young man of Naïn. He was hastily carried out of the city to be buried. Jesus walked up to the bier and apparently had enough time to look at the presumed dead man, observe his breathing, and possibly feel for a pulse. As was the custom at the time to determine death, he called him and gave him the order to get up. With success, as the story describes.

Abstract: Apparent death ICD-10 R09.0

1.16 Jesus Calms a Storm

1.16.1 Original Text (Luke 8:22–25, Mark 4:35–41)

Jesus Calms a Storm (Luke 8:22–25): 22 One day he got into a boat with his disciples, and he said to them, "Let us go across to the other side of the lake." So they set out, 23 and as they sailed he fell asleep. And a windstorm came down on the lake, and they were filling with water and were in danger. 24 And they went and woke him, saying, "Master, Master, we are perishing!" And he awoke and rebuked the wind and the raging waves, and they ceased, and there was a calm. 25 He said to them, "Where is your faith?" And they were afraid, and they marveled, saying to one another, "Who then is this, that he commands even winds and water, and they obey him?".

Jesus Calms a Storm (Mark 4:35–41): 35 On that day, when evening had come, he said to them, "Let us go across to the other side." 36 And leaving the crowd, they took him with them in the boat, just as he was. And other boats were with him. 37 And a great windstorm arose, and the waves were breaking into the boat, so that the boat was already filling. 38 But he was in the stern, asleep on the cushion. And they woke him and said to him, "Teacher, do you not care that we are perishing?" 39 And he awoke and rebuked the wind and said to the sea, "Peace! Be still!" And the wind ceased, and there was a great calm. 40 He said to

[105] "Die Todesfeststellung in der Geschichte der Medizin." MTA Dialog, 22 Nov. 2021, www.mta-dialog.de/artikel/die-todesfeststellung-in-der-geschichte-der-medizin.html.

[106] Autoren der Wikimedia-Projekte. "Scheintod – Wikipedia." 14 Sept. 2004, de.wikipedia.org/w/index.php?title=Scheintod&oldid=217070636.

them, "Why are you so afraid? Have you still no faith?" 41 And they were filled with great fear and said to one another, "Who then is this, that even the wind and the sea obey him?".

1.16.2 Description and Interpretation

Jesus had had a strenuous day and in the evening told his disciples, "let's go to the other side of the lake". A storm came up, and the disciples were afraid because the waves were already crashing into the boat. Jesus, however, was asleep in the boat and did not notice any of this. The disciples woke Jesus up and told him that they were going to sink. Jesus got up and commanded the storm to be calm. Thereupon the wind calmed down, and the waves calmed down. He then reproached his disciples for not having faith and too little confidence. "Why are you so afraid, have you no faith". But the disciples saw the incident as a miracle and wondered what kind of man this was, whom even wind and water obeyed.

The journey apparently went from Capernaum (northwest side of the lake of Galilee) to the east side of the lake. This area is known for **sudden thermal winds** that can be very strong, originating from the surrounding mountains. These strong winds still exist today, which is why it is advertised on the Internet as "Europe's most popular region for wind surfers".[107] In the Bible it is described that a sudden storm arose and the disciples who were sitting in the boat were very afraid. The danger might not have been that great, because the disciples were not alone, other boats were accompanying them (Mark 4:36) and there is no panic reaction described in the other boats in the Bible.

It is well known that winds do not always blow evenly there. Wind gusts are a well-known phenomenon that everyone has experienced at least once. On the homepage of the German Weather Service, wind gusts are defined as "sudden and brief increases in wind speed". In this case, the measured 10-min average must be exceeded by at least 10 knots (5 m/s) within a few seconds. Mostly gusts are brief, lasting usually no longer than 10–20 min.[108]

One of the causes of gusts is that the wind blows at different strengths at different altitudes. At high altitudes, the wind speed is greater Now, when the air near the ground heats up during the day, warm air rises. To compensate, the air must sink in other places. This effect causes an exchange of the air masses of lower and upper air layers. This exchange effect causes the wind speed and gusts to increase as the ground warms during the day. Then, in the evening and at night, the wind often abates rapidly.

The crossing began toward evening, apparently at a time when air mixing was still relatively strong. The evening decrease in wind speed down to calmness is a normal

---

107 "Israel: See Genetareth." Www.surf-magazin, 5 Oct. 2018, www.surf-magazin.de/reisen/naher_osten/israel-see-genetareth.

108 "Wetter und Klima - Deutscher Wetterdienst - Windböen - Unwetterklimatologie: Extreme Windböen." 25 Nov. 2021, www.dwd.de/DE/leistungen/unwetterklima/windboeen/windboeen.html.

phenomenon. In the vernacular, the expression "**the wind dropped**" is often used. If there were gusts of wind during the crossing of the Sea of Galilee and Jesus was asleep, one can well imagine that the disciples did not wake Jesus up immediately, but waited a little longer until their fear was so great that they decided to wake him up after all. A time that might have taken about 10–20 min. After they woke Jesus up and he "commanded" the wind to be calm, he scolded them for their timidity. This was not really a miracle but rather a normal phenomenon, namely that **gusty down drafts spontaneously decrease towards evening**, cannot be proven to have applied here, but is in any case more likely than a miracle.

Abstract: Temporal normal natural phenomenon.

1.17 Jesus Heals Two Blind Men (The Healing of Two Blind Men)

1.17.1 Original Text (Matthew 9:27–31)

Jesus Heals Two Blind Men (Matthew 9:27–3): 27 And as Jesus passed on from there, two blind men followed him, crying aloud, "Have mercy on us, Son of David." 28 When he entered the house, the blind men came to him, and Jesus said to them, "Do you believe that I am able to do this?" They said to him, "Yes, Lord." 29 Then he touched their eyes, saying, "According to your faith be it done to you." 30 And their eyes were opened. And Jesus sternly warned them, "See that no one knows about it." 31 But they went away and spread his fame through all that district.

1.17.2 Description and Interpretation

Two blind men, noticing that Jesus is near them, call out to him and ask Jesus to heal them. Jesus asks them, "do you believe that I can do this?" They answered him that they believe so. In response, Jesus touched their eyes and says, "let it be done as you believe". Thereupon their eyes were opened. But Jesus instructed them not to tell anyone about it. But they did not comply and told everyone in the whole region.

Jesus healed several blind people during his life. The explanation for this is probably the same as in the case described in Matthew 20:30. Interestingly, Jesus does not claim that he will heal them, but only asks them if they believe that they could be helped. After touching their eyes, he does not tell them that they can see again, but only that they will be helped as they believe. Thus, the success is no longer up to him, but up to the people concerned. If they see, then they have healed themselves. If they do not see, their faith was not strong enough. If it is a psychogenic blindness or psychogenic visual impairment,[109] he can expect to succeed, if not, the blame of failure is not on him, because their faith was simply not strong enough.

This is a clever strategy of Jesus to mobilize self-healing forces. What the blind may really have suffered from cannot be deduced from the short biblical text, since there is no close description of the nature of the blindness. However, the rapid success points to psychogenic blindness.

Abstract: psychogenic blindness or visual impairment (ICD-10: F44.6).

1.18 Jesus Heals a Man Unable to Speak

1.18.1 Original Text (Luke 11:14–16; Matthew 9:32–34)

Jesus and Beelzebul (Luke 11:14–16): 14 Now he was casting out a demon that was mute. When the demon had gone out, the mute man spoke, and the people marveled. 15 But some of them said, "He casts out demons by Beelzebul, the prince of demons," 16 while others, to test him, kept seeking from him a sign from heaven.

Jesus Heals a Man Unable to Speak (Matthew 9:32–34): 32 As they were going away, behold, a demon-oppressed man who was mute was brought to him. 33 And when the demon had been cast out, the mute man spoke. And the crowds marveled, saying, "Never was anything like this seen in Israel." 34 But the Pharisees said, "He casts out demons by the prince of demons."

1.18.2 Description and Interpretation

A mute man, who was supposedly possessed by a demon, was brought to Jesus. Jesus cast out the demon, whereupon the mute could speak again. Since no one could explain how such a thing was possible, the Pharisees claimed that Jesus himself must be in contact with the demons, otherwise he could not perform such exorcisms.

Mutism is a symptom that is often associated with other mental illnesses and often begins in childhood after psychological trauma.[110] The affected person could speak but does not or speaks only with certain people or in certain situations, so-called **selective mutism**.[111] In adulthood, this symptom is also called **psychogenic**

---

[109] Dattilo M, Biousse V, Bruce BB, Newman NJ. Functional and simulated visual loss. Handb Clin Neurol. 2016;139:329–341. doi: https://doi.org/10.1016/B978-0-12-801772-2.00029-1. PMID: 27719853.

[110] Hua A, Major N. Selective mutism. Curr Opin Pediatr. 2016 Feb;28(1):114–20. doi: https://doi.org/10.1097/MOP.0000000000000300. PMID: 26709680.

[111] Rozenek EB, Orlof W, Nowicka ZM, Wilczyńska K, Waszkiewicz N. Selective mutism—an overview of the condition and etiology: is the absence of speech just the tip of the iceberg? Psychiatr Pol. 2020 Apr 30;54(2):333–349. English, Polish. doi: https://doi.org/10.12740/PP/OnlineFirst/108503. Epub 2020 Apr 30. PMID: 32772064.

(hysterical, functional) aphonia. As a cause, psychiatric diseases like depression or schizophrenia are possible.[112] But also emotional conflicts in the context of a neurotic conflict processing disorder (with conversion neurotic hysterical symptom formation) can lead to mutism. Since the Bible states that the man in question was possessed by a demon, it is most likely that he suffered from **psychosis** or **obsessive–compulsive disorder**. These disorders are usually accompanied by the very peculiar behaviour of the affected person and may be associated with selective mutism.[113]

Abstract: Mutism (ICD-10: 94.9) or aphonia (ICD-10: F44.4 or R49.1 or DSM-5 key: F44.4).

1.19 Jesus Heals a Man with a Demon (Healing of the Possessed Man from Gerasa)

1.19.1 Original Text (Luke 8:26–39; Mark 5:1–20; Matthew 8:28–34)

Jesus Heals a Man with a Demon (Luke 8:26–39): 26 Then they sailed to the country of the Gerasenes, which is opposite Galilee. 27 When Jesus had stepped out on land, there met him a man from the city who had demons. For a long time he had worn no clothes, and he had not lived in a house but among the tombs. 28 When he saw Jesus, he cried out and fell down before him and said with a loud voice, "What have you to do with me, Jesus, Son of the Most High God? I beg you, do not torment me." 29 For he had commanded the unclean spirit to come out of the man. (For many a time it had seized him. He was kept under guard and bound with chains and shackles, but he would break the bonds and be driven by the demon into the desert.) 30 Jesus then asked him, "What is your name?" And he said, "Legion," for many demons had entered him. 31 And they begged him not to command them to depart into the abyss. 32 Now a large herd of pigs was feeding there on the hillside, and they begged him to let them enter these. So he gave them permission. 33 Then the demons came out of the man and entered the pigs, and the herd rushed down the steep bank into the lake and drowned. 34 When the herdsmen saw what had happened, they fled and told it in the city and in the country. 35 Then people went out to see what had happened, and they came to Jesus and found the man from whom the demons had gone, sitting at the feet of Jesus, clothed and in his right mind, and they were afraid. 36 And those who had seen it told them how the demon-possessed man had been healed. 37 Then all the people of the surrounding country of the Gerasenes asked him to depart from them, for they were seized with great fear. So he got into the boat and returned. 38 The man from whom the demons had gone begged that he might be with him, but Jesus sent him away, saying, 39 "Return to your home, and declare how much God has done for you." And he went away, proclaiming throughout the whole city how much Jesus had done for him.

---

[112] Naqvi Y, Gupta V. Functional Voice Disorders. 2021 Oct 4. In: StatPearls [Internet]. Treasure Island (FL): StatPearls Publishing; 2021 Jan. PMID: 33085329.

[113] Vani P, Nadella RK, Viswanath B, Jain S. Mutism as a component of obsessive-compulsive symptoms in patients with schizophrenia: A report of two cases. Asian J Psychiatr. 2020 Dec;54:102337. doi: https://doi.org/10.1016/j.ajp.2020.102337. Epub 2020 Aug 6. PMID: 32795956.

Jesus Heals a Man with a Demon (Mark 5:1–20): 1 They came to the other side of the sea, to the country of the Gerasenes. 2 And when Jesus had stepped out of the boat, immediately there met him out of the tombs a man with an unclean spirit. 3 He lived among the tombs. And no one could bind him anymore, not even with a chain, 4 for he had often been bound with shackles and chains, but he wrenched the chains apart, and he broke the shackles in pieces. No one had the strength to subdue him. 5 Night and day among the tombs and on the mountains he was always crying out and cutting himself with stones. 6 And when he saw Jesus from afar, he ran and fell down before him. 7 And crying out with a loud voice, he said, "What have you to do with me, Jesus, Son of the Most High God? I adjure you by God, do not torment me." 8 For he was saying to him, "Come out of the man, you unclean spirit!" 9 And Jesus asked him, "What is your name?" He replied, "My name is Legion, for we are many." 10 And he begged him earnestly not to send them out of the country. 11 Now a great herd of pigs was feeding there on the hillside, 12 and they begged him, saying, "Send us to the pigs; let us enter them." 13 So he gave them permission. And the unclean spirits came out and entered the pigs; and the herd, numbering about two thousand, rushed down the steep bank into the sea and drowned in the sea. 14 The herdsmen fled and told it in the city and in the country. And people came to see what it was that had happened. 15 And they came to Jesus and saw the demon-possessed man, the one who had had the legion, sitting there, clothed and in his right mind, and they were afraid. 16 And those who had seen it described to them what had happened to the demon-possessed man and to the pigs. 17 And they began to beg Jesus to depart from their region. 18 As he was getting into the boat, the man who had been possessed with demons begged him that he might be with him. 19 And he did not permit him but said to him, "Go home to your friends and tell them how much the Lord has done for you, and how he has had mercy on you." 20 And he went away and began to proclaim in the Decapolis how much Jesus had done for him, and everyone marveled.

Jesus Heals Two Men with Demons (Matthew 8:28–34): 28 And when he came to the other side, to the country of the Gadarenes, two demon-possessed men met him, coming out of the tombs, so fierce that no one could pass that way. 29 And behold, they cried out, "What have you to do with us, O Son of God? Have you come here to torment us before the time?" 30 Now a herd of many pigs was feeding at some distance from them. 31 And the demons begged him, saying, "If you cast us out, send us away into the herd of pigs." 32 And he said to them, "Go." So they came out and went into the pigs, and behold, the whole herd rushed down the steep bank into the sea and drowned in the waters. 33 The herdsmen fled, and going into the city they told everything, especially what had happened to the demon-possessed men. 34 And behold, all the city came out to meet Jesus, and when they saw him, they begged him to leave their region.

1.19.2 Description and Interpretation

Jesus comes to the area of Gerasa in a region near a lake. There lived an apparently mentally ill man who could no longer be integrated into normal society and was therefore excluded from their community by the local villagers. This meant that he no longer had a place to live. He sought shelter in the burial grounds located near his village. Not even clothes were given to him by the villagers. Possibly a second "madman" joined him. Thus, they eked out a poor existence at the cemetery, where they at least had a roof over their heads in the old burial grounds.

The "crazy man" was afraid of the people, and the people were afraid of him. Whenever new people came near him, the encounter was characterized by fear and aggression. So it was apparently when Jesus came to this area and the mad man rushed at him screaming. Jesus met him with composure and mastered the whole situation by keeping calm. The only problem was that at the end of this aggressive encounter, numerous pigs panicked and drowned in the nearby lake. This spectacle must have been very impressive because it was reported by three evangelists in unison. Added to this excitement, there was economic damage. Allegedly, 2,000 pigs drowned in the lake during this incident. It should therefore not be surprising that the local population asked Jesus, who was of course "to blame" for everything, to leave the country again as quickly as possible.

How could it happen that a whole herd of pigs suddenly panics, runs away and plunges into the water? The simplest explanation would be that **animals can also be afraid and panic**. In North America, some Indian tribes have even used this effect for "**panic hunting**". Entire herds of buffalo were driven in the direction of a precipice or a frozen lake so that the animals could crash or break into the ice and then be easily killed.[114] In any case, animals sense fear emanating from the environment and react to it. Anyone who has ever experienced what goes on when two dog owners get into a tussle with their leashed dogs can confirm how quickly aggression is transferred from the owners to the dogs.

That pigs seem to display a special empathy towards humans and even develop feelings that we would call empathy, has been shown in recent studies.[115] Also, in our language, expressions like "to have animal fear" have become established, which suggests that this empathic capacity of animals and especially pigs has been felt by us humans for a long time.

So the incident might have happened as follows: An apparently mentally ill person, who had already experienced much suffering from the villagers living nearby, sees a new unknown crowd (Jesus and his companions) approaching him. He runs towards Jesus, excited and shouting because he is afraid of the arriving group of people. The fear can be explained in so far as he had experienced evil from "normal" people again and again in the past. He had even had to endure torture and bondage from the "normal" people. In addition to this, mentally ill people perceive dangerous situations in an exaggerated way, so that a fear quickly turns into panic reactions.[116] Given this, however, the probability is high that **also the pigs could panic and run away**. One may assume that the pigs otherwise experienced the "madman" as "normal" i.e. without panic, so something very dangerous must have happened suddenly, and therefore they followed their **escape reflex**. Unfortunately, the escape ended in the water, so they drowned. Pigs are not known to be good swimmers. However, **panicked pigs are not "evidence of demons that have passed from humans to animals"**. Humans also do completely crazy things in fear situations. So also the shepherds were obviously afraid and ran away ("The shepherds fled and told it in the city and

[114] www.indianerwww.de. "Die Indianer Nordamerikas - Jagd- und Fangmethoden." www.indianerwww.de, 21 Dec. 2001, www.indianerwww.de/indian/jagdmethoden.htm.

[115] Kollman Barabara: Auch Schweine kennen Mitgefühl, Welt.de 2015; https://www.welt.de/wissenschaft/umwelt/article137042031/Auch-Schweine-kennen-Mitgefuehl.html.

[116] Goodwin R, Davidson L. Panic attacks in psychosis. Acta Psychiatr Scand. 2002 Jan;105(1):14–9. doi: https://doi.org/10.1034/j.1600-0447.2002._10424.x. PMID: 12086220.

in the villages. Then the people rushed to see what had happened"). But neither in humans nor in animals do these panic reactions have anything to do with demons or evil spirits.

Let us return to the first part of this story. The Bible tells in relative detail about this strange and allegedly "possessed" man. He lived in tombs, i.e. **he lived in social isolation**, secluded from the rest of society at the cemetery, where already under normal circumstances nobody would dare to go at night. After he had been maltreated several times with shackles and chains, he could be halfway safe there, at least at night, not to be attacked by the "normal" people. The fact that he repeatedly wore through the foot shackles is a highly normal reaction of a shackled person. The sentence "**no one was able to overcome him**" shows that the society surrounding him repeatedly tried to do violence to the "possessed" man and that he successfully defended himself against it. In general, he seemed to be afraid of people, which should not be particularly surprising given his past history. This also explains the aggressive behaviour, the behaviour that this poor man displayed. He became, so to speak, a "**fear-biter**" (a dog that bites other, more powerful, dogs because it is frightened).[117] Whenever someone came near him, he showed himself aggressively. Thus, people finally did not dare to come near him. He also showed repeated self-harming behaviour when he repeatedly hit his own head with a stone. Such behaviour represents a well-known symptom of mentally ill people with **borderline disorder**.[118] Also, today we know people who inflict pain on themselves (e.g. deep scratching, carving). This behaviour is known as **body-focused repetitive behaviour disorder**.[119] It is believed that the self-inflicted pain triggers a release of endorphins that provide temporary relief. Therefore, such people experience a sense of relief from pain, while "normal" people experience a sense of distress from pain.[120]

Nowadays, a psychiatrist would determine several psychiatric diagnoses or make the collective diagnosis of "polymorphic psychosis" with the following additional diagnoses:

- **Dissociative personality disorder, with a lack of learning ability** ("again, and again he screamed and harassed other people") and apparently **violent behaviour** ("everyone was afraid to pass there"). Dissociative personality disorder is now often seen in criminal people who had traumatic experiences in early childhood and grew up in very poor environmental conditions.[121]

---

[117] Hoffmann, Sven Olaf. "»Menschliche Angstbeißer«." in Persönlichkeitsstörungen Theorie und Praxis, Klett-Cotta, Schattauer, ptt, vol. 16, no. 4, 2012, pp. 225–31, https://elibrary.klett-cotta.de/article/99.120110/ptt-16-4-225.

[118] Colle L, Hilviu D, Rossi R, Garbarini F, Fossataro C. Self-Harming and Sense of Agency in Patients With Borderline Personality Disorder. Front Psychiatry. 2020 May 29;11:449. doi: https://doi.org/10.3389/fpsyt.2020.00449. PMID: 32547429; PMCID: PMC7273851.

[119] Grant JE, Stein DJ. Body-focused repetitive behavior disorders in ICD-11. Braz J Psychiatry. 2014;36 Suppl 1:59–64. doi: https://doi.org/10.1590/1516-4446-2013-1228. PMID: 25388613.

[120] Own clinical experience, not published.

[121] Glenn AL, Johnson AK, Raine A. Antisocial personality disorder: a current review. Curr Psychiatry Rep. 2013 Dec;15(12):427. doi: https://doi.org/10.1007/s11920-013-0427-7. PMID: 24249521.

- **Emotionally unstable personality disorder** is another characteristic of the person described. He had symptoms of **impulsivity type** with lack of control of his own aggressive behaviour such as outbursts of rage or loud shouting (rioting) as well as symptoms of unstable personality disorder of **borderline type** in which the control of emotions is strongly limited.[122] The smallest occasions (arrival of Jesus and his disciples) can immediately lead to long-lasting and excessive reactions in these people. Also, the **self-injurious behaviour**[123] is often seen in this form of mood disorder. Nowadays, affected people no longer knock themselves on the head with a stone, but carve their forearms or get full tattoos all over their body. Also, here physical neglect, lack of caregivers, a profoundly changing emotional world and neglect can be found. Frequently these people have experienced violence and sexual abuse in their early childhood.

After this incident, people from the surrounding area came and saw the "**demon-possessed man sitting with Jesus, normally clothed and in his right mind**". The fact that the man was normally clothed indicates that some time must have passed. Followers of Jesus must have procured clothes, and Jesus apparently had enough time to calm the possessed man and gain his trust. However, this may not have been the only reason that the possessed man appeared normal and sane again. **Patients with emotionally unstable personality disorder typically present with highly changeable emotions**. For example, they may be rowdy at one time, only to return to relatively normal behaviour the next second. This disorder, also referred to as borderline type unstable emotional disorder, is also found in many couple relationships, which would be popularly referred to as "love-hate" relationships. Hot love turns into blind hatred in a flash, and then turns back into uncritical admiration. But this also has nothing to do with "unclean spirits", but rather points to a **disturbed impulse control**, as often occurs in disorders of the serotonergic nervous system. Also, the possessed man had suddenly found a great affection for Jesus and wanted to stay with him. "When he got into the boat, the man who had previously been possessed by demons asked him that he might be with him". Jesus was wise enough to forbid him. Jesus did not permit him, but said, "Go home and tell your family all that the Lord has done for you and how he has had mercy on you"!

---

[122] Gunderson JG, Herpertz SC, Skodol AE, Torgersen S, Zanarini MC. Borderline personality disorder. Nat Rev Dis Primers. 2018 May 24;4:18029. doi: https://doi.org/10.1038/nrdp.2018.29. PMID: 29795363.

[123] Huisman S, Mulder P, Kuijk J, Kerstholt M, van Eeghen A, Leenders A, van Balkom I, Oliver C, Piening S, Hennekam R. Self-injurious behavior. Neurosci Biobehav Rev. 2018 Jan;84:483–491. doi: https://doi.org/10.1016/j.neubiorev.2017.02.027. Epub 2017 Jul 8. PMID: 28694012.

Abstract: Polymorphic psychosis (ICD-10 F23.1), dissociative personality disorder (ICD-10 F44.7) and emotionally unstable personality disorder of impulsivity type (ICD-10 F 60.2) and borderline type (ICD-10 F 60.3), anxiety disorder (ICD-10 F41.9) and panic disorder (ICD-10 F41.0), post-traumatic stress disorder (ICD-10 F05.).

1.20 Jesus Heals a Woman and Jairus's Daughter (A Girl Restored to Life and a Woman Healed)

1.20.1 Original Text (Luke 8:41–56; Mark 5:21–43; Matthew 9:18–26)

Jesus Heals a Woman and Jairus's Daughter (Luke 8:41–56): 40 Now when Jesus returned, the crowd welcomed him, for they were all waiting for him. 41 And there came a man named Jairus, who was a ruler of the synagogue. And falling at Jesus' feet, he implored him to come to his house, 42 for he had an only daughter, about twelve years of age, and she was dying. As Jesus went, the people pressed around him. 43 And there was a woman who had had a discharge of blood for twelve years, and though she had spent all her living on physicians, she could not be healed by anyone. 44 She came up behind him and touched the fringe of his garment, and immediately her discharge of blood ceased. 45 And Jesus said, "Who was it that touched me?" When all denied it, Peter said, "Master, the crowds surround you and are pressing in on you!" 46 But Jesus said, "Someone touched me, for I perceive that power has gone out from me." 47 And when the woman saw that she was not hidden, she came trembling, and falling down before him declared in the presence of all the people why she had touched him, and how she had been immediately healed. 48 And he said to her, "Daughter, your faith has made you well; go in peace." 49 While he was still speaking, someone from the ruler's house came and said, "Your daughter is dead; do not trouble the Teacher any more." 50 But Jesus on hearing this answered him, "Do not fear; only believe, and she will be well." 51 And when he came to the house, he allowed no one to enter with him, except Peter and John and James, and the father and mother of the child. 52 And all were weeping and mourning for her, but he said, "Do not weep, for she is not dead but sleeping." 53 And they laughed at him, knowing that she was dead. 54 But taking her by the hand he called, saying, "Child, arise." 55 And her spirit returned, and she got up at once. And he directed that something should be given her to eat. 56 And her parents were amazed, but he charged them to tell no one what had happened.

Jesus Heals a Woman and Jairus's Daughter (Mark 5:21–43): 21 And when Jesus had crossed again in the boat to the other side, a great crowd gathered about him, and he was beside the sea. 22 Then came one of the rulers of the synagogue, Jairus by name, and seeing him, he fell at his feet 23 and implored him earnestly, saying, "My little daughter is at the point of death. Come and lay your hands on her, so that she may be made well and live." 24 And he went with him. And a great crowd followed him and thronged about him. 25 And there was a woman who had had a discharge of blood for twelve years, 26 and who had suffered much under many physicians, and had spent all that she had, and was no better but rather grew worse. 27 She had heard the reports about Jesus and came up behind him in the crowd and touched his garment. 28 For she said, "If I touch even his garments, I will be made well." 29 And immediately the flow of blood dried up, and she felt in her body that she was healed of her disease. 30 And Jesus, perceiving in himself that power had gone out from him, immediately turned about in the crowd and said, "Who touched my garments?" 31 And his disciples said to him, "You see the crowd pressing around you, and yet you say, 'Who touched me?'" 32 And he looked around to see who had done it. 33 But the woman, knowing what had happened to her, came in fear and trembling and fell down before him and told him the whole truth. 34 And he said to her, "Daughter, your faith has made you well; go in peace, and be healed of your disease." 35 While he was still speaking, there came from the ruler's house some who said, "Your daughter is dead. Why trouble the Teacher any further?" 36 But overhearing[5] what they said, Jesus said to the ruler of the synagogue, "Do not fear, only believe." 37 And he allowed no one to follow him except Peter and James and John the brother of James. 38 They came to the house of the ruler of the synagogue, and Jesus[6] saw a commotion, people weeping and wailing loudly. 39 And when he had entered, he said to them, "Why are you making a commotion and weeping? The child is not dead but sleeping." 40 And they laughed at him. But he put them all outside and took the child's father and mother and those who were with him and went in where the child was. 41 Taking her by the hand he said to her, "Talitha cumi," which means, "Little girl, I say to you, arise." 42 And immediately the girl got up and began walking (for she was twelve years of age), and they were immediately overcome with amazement. 43 And he strictly charged them that no one should know this, and told them to give her something to eat.

A Girl Restored to Life and a Woman Healed (Matthew 9:18–26): 18 While he was saying these things to them, behold, a ruler came in and knelt before him, saying, "My daughter has just died, but come and lay your hand on her, and she will live." 19 And Jesus rose and followed him, with his disciples. 20 And behold, a woman who had suffered from a discharge of blood for twelve years came up behind him and touched the fringe of his garment, 21 for she said to herself, "If I only touch his garment, I will be made well." 22 Jesus turned, and seeing her he said, "Take heart, daughter; your faith has made you well." And instantly[4] the woman was made well. 23 And when Jesus came to the ruler's house and saw the flute players and the crowd making a commotion, 24 he said, "Go away, for the girl is not dead but sleeping." And they laughed at him. 25 But when the crowd had been put outside, he went in and took her by the hand, and the girl arose. 26 And the report of this went through all that district.

1.20.2 Description and Interpretation

A synagogue ruler, named Jaïrus, came to Jesus, threw himself at his feet and asked him to come to his home and help him. His 12-year-old daughter was dying. While Jesus was on his way there, a miraculous healing of a woman occurred. While Jesus was dealing with this woman, the servants came from the synagogue ruler's house and reported that his daughter had died in the meantime. Jesus should save himself the trip there, because it would already be too late. In any case, nothing could be done. Then Jesus told the synagogue ruler not to be afraid and went to the ruler's house anyway. Once there, he saw the relatives already loudly lamenting the girl's death. Jesus went to the girl and said to the bystanders that the child was not dead, but only asleep. The people present there laughed at Jesus and mocked him. Jesus sent everyone out and went with the child's parents closer to the bed of the one who was supposedly dead. He held the daughter's hand and said, "Girl, I tell you, get up". Thereupon the girl got up and showed herself quite alive. Jesus instructed the parents to give her something to eat and not to tell anyone about it.

This story is actually two different miracles, which are always told together, because they coincided in time. Both incidents have, however, nothing to do with each other. Here, only the raising from the dead of the girl is interpreted. The miraculous healing from the continuous flow of blood is discussed in case No. 21.

In the case of a 12-year-old girl, it can be assumed that she was at the beginning of her sexual maturity. **At the beginning of puberty**, the control of the cycle is still a bit bumpy and **cycles without ovulation occur**[124] again and again. Only with increasing age does a harmonious, regular monthly cycle develop. This is also true for most women today.

Around ovulation there are serious changes not only in hormonal balance but also in breathing control.[125] Women hyperventilate so consistently that it is even possible to determine ovulation by determining the respiratory gases. Appropriate devices for the determination of ovulation by respiratory gas analysis are already in development.[126] However, it is important to know that **hyperventilation**, i.e. breathing too fast or too deeply, can cause massive changes in the electrolyte balance with disturbances in nerve function. This leads to nerve dysfunction and subsequently paralysis. While most women do not feel anything from this **hormone-induced change in breathing**, some girls or young women may experience **panic attacks**, which in turn lead to an increase in hyperventilation. This creates a vicious circle or, in scientific terms, a positive feedback loop: hyperventilation leads to panic attacks, which in turn lead to increased hyperventilation. The anxiety reaction can increase to such an extent that the affected person not only develops increasing **symptoms of paralysis**, but eventually becomes **unconscious, as if appearing dead.**[127] Due to unconsciousness, breathing returns to normal, and it takes time for them to regain consciousness. The whole thing can be quite dramatic and sometimes lasts for a long period of time. Occasionally the affected person even screams and thus transmits their own fear to the bystanders as well. In the past, this reaction was called a hysterical fit and women who had it more often were called "hysterical women". Today, one would speak of panic attacks with hyperventilation syndrome.

An alternative explanation would be an **epileptic seizure, which can also be triggered by hyperventilation.**[128] Again, it is not only the sufferer who feels bad,

---

[124] Carlson LJ, Shaw ND. Development of Ovulatory Menstrual Cycles in Adolescent Girls. J Pediatr Adolesc Gynecol. 2019 Jun;32(3):249–253. doi: https://doi.org/10.1016/j.jpag.2019.02.119. Epub 2019 Feb 14. PMID: 30772499; PMCID: PMC6570576.

[125] Slatkovska L, Jensen D, Davies GA, Wolfe LA. Phasic menstrual cycle effects on the control of breathing in healthy women. Respir Physiol Neurobiol. 2006 Dec;154(3):379–88. doi: https://doi.org/10.1016/j.resp.2006.01.011. Epub 2006 Mar 15. PMID: 16542884.

[126] Hadziomerović D, Moeller KT, Licht P, Hein A, Veitenhansel S, Kusmitsch M, Wildt L. The biphasic pattern of end-expiratory carbon dioxide pressure: a method for identification of the fertile phase of the menstrual cycle. Fertil Steril. 2008 Sep;90(3):731–6. doi: https://doi.org/10.1016/j.fertnstert.2007.06.078. Epub 2007 Oct 23. PMID: 17936278.

[127] Perkin GD, Joseph R. Neurological manifestations of the hyperventilation syndrome. J R Soc Med. 1986 Aug;79(8):448–50. doi: https://doi.org/10.1177/014107688607900805. PMID: 3761286; PMCID: PMC1290412.

[128] Indranada AM, Mullen SA, Duncan R, Berlowitz DJ, Kanaan RAA. The association of panic and hyperventilation with psychogenic non-epileptic seizures: A systematic review and meta-analysis.

but also the bystanders. If sufferers convulse, foam at the mouth and sometimes also scream during the seizure, then these features will particularly cause uproar in the surrounding humans. If the seizure is then over, it may be followed by a **postictal twilight state**, the so-called **Todd's paralysis.**[129] In this case, the person lies limply paralysed with clouding of consciousness on the floor and can easily appear dead.[130] The **twilight state dissolves after some time by itself** and the original state is restored.

Another explanation for the "raising of the synagogue ruler's daughter" would be a so-called **hysterical seizure**, today called a **dissociative seizure**. Obviously, things were already quite dramatic before the supposed death, otherwise the synagogue ruler would not have run to meet Jesus and asked him for help. Such dramatic situations often play out theatrically, especially when they are **"hysterical" episodes**. Such episodes are more common, especially among young women, and they can cause quite a stir.

The term hysteria comes from the Greek because women who had such episodes were believed to have the uterus (hystera) slipping into the neck, where it clogged the throat. This explanation is based on the observation that affected women often feel a "lump in the throat" (globus sensation) at the beginning of such attacks. When children are sad and begin to cry, they typically describe "feeling a lump" in their throat. Today we say conversion neurotic episodes, or panic attacks, are preceded by a (family) quarrel. So the bad conscience of the housemates of this house is an additional factor. When a panic attack develops in the context of a family conflict and the child begins to show signs of paralysis, we frequently see that in such cases the parents call for help. By the time this arrives, everything has miraculously healed itself, and the parents are usually embarrassed to have called for help "for nothing". It must have been the same with Jesus, who, so to speak, represented the function of the "rescuer" at that time.

Jesus recognized quickly that the girl was not dead, but only "sleeping" and/or had clouded consciousness. His sovereign charisma and calmness was the best first aid imaginable in such a case.

Abstract: Unconsciousness (ICD-10 R40.2) in dissociative disorder (ICD-10 F44.8) with hyperventilation syndrome (ICD-10 R06.4).

Seizure. 2018 Jul;59:108–115. doi: https://doi.org/10.1016/j.seizure.2018.05.007. Epub 2018 May 19. PMID: 29787922.

[129] Winsløw F, Meden P, Havsteen IB, Tsiropoulos I. [Todd's paralysis]. Ugeskr Laeger. 2021 Apr 19;183(16):V06200455. Danish. PMID: 33913429.

[130] McClain IJ, Tsai MA, Guardia CF 3rd. Prolonged Postictal Coma in Hemiplegic Migraine: A Case Report. Headache. 2019 Oct;59(9):1641–1642. doi: https://doi.org/10.1111/head.13606. Epub 2019 Jul 24. PMID: 31339554.

1.21 Jesus Heals a Woman with Discharge of Blood

1.21.1 Original Text (Luke 8:43–48; Mark 5:25–34, Matthew 9:18–26)

Jesus Heals a Woman (Luke 8:43–48): 43 And there was a woman who had had a discharge of blood for twelve years, and though she had spent all her living on physicians, she could not be healed by anyone. 44 She came up behind him and touched the fringe of his garment, and immediately her discharge of blood ceased. 45 And Jesus said, "Who was it that touched me?" When all denied it, Peter said, "Master, the crowds surround you and are pressing in on you!" 46 But Jesus said, "Someone touched me, for I perceive that power has gone out from me." 47 And when the woman saw that she was not hidden, she came trembling, and falling down before him declared in the presence of all the people why she had touched him, and how she had been immediately healed. 48 And he said to her, "Daughter, your faith has made you well; go in peace."

Jesus Heals a Woman (Mark 5:25–34): 25 And there was a woman who had had a discharge of blood for twelve years, 26 and who had suffered much under many physicians, and had spent all that she had, and was no better, but rather grew worse. 27 She had heard the reports about Jesus and came up behind him in the crowd and touched his garment. 28 For she said, "If I touch even his garments, I will be made well." 29 And immediately the flow of blood dried up, and she felt in her body that she was healed of her disease. 30 And Jesus, perceiving in himself that power had gone out from him, immediately turned about in the crowd and said, "Who touched my garments?" 31 And his disciples said to him, "You see the crowd pressing around you, and yet you say, 'Who touched me?'" 32 And he looked around to see who had done it. 33 But the woman, knowing what had happened to her, came in fear and trembling and fell down before him and told him the whole truth. 34 And he said to her, "Daughter, your faith has made you well; go in peace, and be healed of your disease."

A Girl Restored to Life and a Woman Healed (Matthew 9:18–26): 18 While he was saying these things to them, behold, a ruler came in and knelt before him, saying, "My daughter has just died, but come and lay your hand on her, and she will live." 19 And Jesus rose and followed him, with his disciples. 20 And behold, a woman who had suffered from a discharge of blood for twelve years came up behind him and touched the fringe of his garment, 21 for she said to herself, "If I only touch his garment, I will be made well." 22 Jesus turned, and seeing her he said, "Take heart, daughter; your faith has made you well." And instantly the woman was made well. 23 And when Jesus came to the ruler's house and saw the flute players and the crowd making a commotion, 24 he said, "Go away, for the girl is not dead but sleeping." And they laughed at him. 25 But when the crowd had been put outside, he went in and took her by the hand, and the girl arose. 26 And the report of this went through all that district.

1.21.2 Description and Interpretation

When Jesus was on his way to a synagogue ruler named Jaïrus to save his daughter who was dying, he was surrounded by a crowd. Among others, there was a woman who had been suffering from continuous menstrual bleeding ("discharge of blood") for 12 years. She had been to many doctors because of it and had spent all her money. But no doctor could help her. Now the only hope left for her was to be miraculously healed by Jesus. She approached Jesus and touched him. Jesus noticed the touch, stopped and asked "who touched me". At first, no one dared admit to the touch, and the woman in question hoped that she would remain unrecognized in the crowd. Jesus looked around, searching for the person who had touched him. Then the woman was afraid and came forward and told the reason for the touch. In doing so, she said publicly that she had been suffering from constant bleeding for years and was convinced that by touching Jesus she would receive healing from her unstoppable bleeding. She also said that her bleeding stopped immediately with the touch. Jesus answered her, "Your faith has saved you, go in peace, you shall be healed from your suffering".

The story of the woman with the flow of blood, who has been making years of pilgrimages from doctor to doctor, spending her entire fortune, could also occur in modern times. Even today, there are numerous patients with psychosomatic illnesses who go "doctor shopping" and spend a fortune in the process. Mostly without success, because either the patients cannot accept the diagnoses and the accompanying therapies, or the doctor does not recognize the psychological cause of the complaints. In any case, this is a common phenomenon that has apparently existed for thousands of years. Anyway, this is the first description of a "doctor shopping phenomenon".[131]

Heavy discharge of blood (hypermenorrhea, menorrhagia) is a sign that almost every woman knows, either because she has been affected by it herself or because she knows someone who has been affected by it. Very often, the heavy flow of blood is accompanied by other symptoms such as **menstrual pain (dysmenorrhea), breast tenderness (mastodynia) and mood swings (dysphoria)**. This symptom complex is referred to by gynaecologists as **premenstrual syndrome (PMS)**[132] or, if mood swings are predominant, as **premenstrual dysphoric syndrome (PMDS)**.[133]

One of the causes of such bleeding abnormalities may be a hormonal imbalance between oestrogens and luteal hormones (progestins). This is usually a relative deficiency of luteal hormones in relation to oestrogen action. While today this imbalance is mainly caused by **oestrogen dominance**, in the past it was rather the result of a **luteal hormone deficiency**. Oestrogen dominance could have existed in the woman in question because she had already been to numerous doctors. Even then, doctors and alternative practitioners treated bleeding abnormalities with herbs and plants that contain abundant phytoestrogens. These include monk's pepper, red clover, pomegranate, and other plants that exert oestrogen-like effects in a woman's body and can worsen many a bleeding disorder. A deficiency of corpus luteum hormone

[131] Sansone RA, Sansone LA. Doctor shopping: a phenomenon of many themes. Innov Clin Neurosci. 2012 Nov;9(11–12):42–6. PMID: 23346518; PMCID: PMC3552465.

[132] Ryu A, Kim TH. Premenstrual syndrome: A mini review. Maturitas. 2015 Dec;82(4):436–40. doi: https://doi.org/10.1016/j.maturitas.2015.08.010. Epub 2015 Aug 28. PMID: 26351143.

[133] Hantsoo L, Epperson CN. Premenstrual Dysphoric Disorder: Epidemiology and Treatment. Curr Psychiatry Rep. 2015 Nov;17(11):87. doi: https://doi.org/10.1007/s11920-015-0628-3. PMID: 26377947; PMCID: PMC4890701.

occurs mainly in the case of insufficient function of the corpus luteum in the ovary (corpus luteum insufficiency)[134] and in the case of psychological stress.[135]

But let's stay with the natural regulation of the corpus luteum hormone: The corpus luteum hormone, progesterone, is normally produced after ovulation in the corpus luteum of the ovary. If there is no ovulation (so-called anovulatory cycles), there is no or insufficient formation of the corpus luteum hormone. As a result, the oestrogen effect, which has led to a strong build-up of the uterine mucosa in the first half of the cycle, cannot be reversed. More blood must therefore be bled off during the next menstrual bleeding. This results in the symptom of hypermenorrhea or **heavy menstrual bleeding.**[136] If a coagulation disorder then exists at the same time, such menstrual bleeding can become extremely heavy. In the case of recurrent anovulatory cycles, which occur particularly often shortly before the menopause, the heavy blood loss can lead to pronounced anaemia. This blood loss is even more pronounced if the affected woman also has a (congenital) coagulation disorder.[137] The affected women are then regularly highly symptomatic, although nowadays, the symptoms are usually attributed to the subsequent iron deficiency. However, the iron deficiency is always only a consequence and never a cause of this phenomenon.[138]

Some genetic diseases occur more frequently in the Jewish population. Among them is a disease associated with an increased tendency to bleed, known as haemophilia C (factor XI deficiency). Possibly, in the case of the woman described in the Bible, there was not only a stress-related bleeding disorder, but also a coagulation disorder, which aggravated the whole affair.

But how can a "miracle healing" occur in such a case with increased discharge of blood? Essential for the healing was the touch of Jesus, or rather his clothes, by the woman. If the woman experiences an **improvement "at the moment of the touch"**, what could have been the cause for the stopping of the discharge of blood? The answer to this question could be the **phenomenon of oxytocin release**. Oxytocin is a hormone that causes uterine contractions and thus a kind of "closure" of the blood vessels. During birth, it causes such strong contractions of the uterus that the child is expelled from the womb. Subsequently, it causes the closure of the blood vessels

---

[134] Dawood MY. Corpus luteal insufficiency. Curr Opin Obstet Gynecol. 1994 Apr;6(2):121–7. PMID: 8193250.

[135] Rafique N, Al-Sheikh MH. Prevalence of menstrual problems and their association with psychological stress in young female students studying health sciences. Saudi Med J. 2018 Jan;39(1):67–73. doi: https://doi.org/10.15537/smj.2018.1.21438. PMID: 29332111; PMCID: PMC5885123.

[136] Jewson M, Purohit P, Lumsden MA. Progesterone and abnormal uterine bleeding/menstrual disorders. Best Pract Res Clin Obstet Gynaecol. 2020 Nov;69:62–73. doi: https://doi.org/10.1016/j.bpobgyn.2020.05.004. Epub 2020 Jun 5. PMID: 32698992.

[137] Djambas Khayat C, Gouider E, von Mackensen S, Abdul Kadir R. Heavy menstrual bleeding in women with inherited bleeding disorders. Haemophilia. 2020 Apr;26 Suppl 3:16–19. doi: https://doi.org/10.1111/hae.13888. PMID: 32356352.

[138] Mansour D, Hofmann A, Gemzell-Danielsson K. A Review of Clinical Guidelines on the Management of Iron Deficiency and Iron-Deficiency Anemia in Women with Heavy Menstrual Bleeding. Adv Ther. 2021 Jan;38(1):201–225. doi: https://doi.org/10.1007/s12325-020-01564-y. Epub 2020 Nov 27. PMID: 33247314; PMCID: PMC7695235.

in the uterus and the expulsion of the afterbirth.[139] Thus, it ensures that the birthing mother does not bleed to death.

However, oxytocin is not only produced during the birth phase. It is also produced more frequently after birth, during breastfeeding. When the mother breastfeeds her child, oxytocin is released more frequently, causing slight contractions of the uterus. This is also perceived as pleasant and thus leads to a bonding reaction between mother and child.[140] The same effect can also be triggered by mechanical stimulation of the nipples, and can thus also cause bonding reactions in the sexual partner. Skin contact (or fur contact in the case of animals), fondling and kissing also lead to increased release of oxytocin, which is why this hormone is also often referred to as the "cuddle hormone".[141] Oxytocin is also released during orgasm in both women and men, and thus also causes social bonding in couples who have a fulfilling sex life. In women, oxytocin also causes rhythmic uterine contractions in this case, further intensifying the orgasmic experience. After this overview of the most important effects of oxytocin, its effect on the coagulation system should be emphasized. Oxytocin not only leads to the constriction of blood vessels and thus to haemostasis, but also has a direct influence on coagulation. That is why today, oxytocin is prescribed in the form of a nasal spray for some forms of haemophilia (diseases with bleeding tendency).

After this digression about the effects of oxytocin, it is important to know how the release of oxytocin can occur. Birth, breastfeeding, caressing, kissing, nipple stimulation, and orgasm we have already learned about as stimuli for oxytocin release. Just **thoughts, short touches, erotic fantasies or merely the sight of a face of an attractive person**[142] **can lead to an increased release of oxytocin**. Thus, it is easy to imagine that in the case of the woman described in the Bible, a massive release of oxytocin was triggered by Jesus' touch alone, resulting in uterine contractions and activation of the blood clotting system. If the oxytocin release is preceded by high oestrogen exposure, e.g., from phyto-estrogens, the uterine contractions are particularly strong. Eating dates also seems to promote oxytocin release, which is why even today Muslim women eat dates (Phoenix dactylifera Linn) before giving birth as a "labour-promoting agent".[143]

---

139 Maggi M, Baldi E, Susini T. Hormonal and local regulation of uterine activity during parturition: Part I—The oxytocin system. J Endocrinol Invest. 1994 Oct;17(9):739–56. doi: https://doi.org/10.1007/BF03347771. PMID: 7868820.

140 Jones C, Barrera I, Brothers S, Ring R, Wahlestedt C. Oxytocin and social functioning. Dialogues Clin Neurosci. 2017 Jun;19(2):193–201. doi: https://doi.org/10.31887/DCNS.2017.19.2/cjones. PMID: 28867943; PMCID: PMC5573563.

141 Carter CS, Kenkel WM, MacLean EL, Wilson SR, Perkeybile AM, Yee JR, Ferris CF, Nazarloo HP, Porges SW, Davis JM, Connelly JJ, Kingsbury MA. Is Oxytocin "Nature's Medicine"? Pharmacol Rev. 2020 Oct;72(4):829–861. doi: https://doi.org/10.1124/pr.120.019398. PMID: 32912963; PMCID: PMC7495339.

142 Proverbio AM. Sex differences in social cognition: The case of face processing. J Neurosci Res. 2017 Jan 2;95(1–2):222–234. doi: https://doi.org/10.1002/jnr.23817. PMID: 27870403.

143 Vayalil PK. Date fruits (Phoenix dactylifera Linn): an emerging medicinal food. Crit Rev Food Sci Nutr. 2012;52(3):249–71. doi: https://doi.org/10.1080/10408398.2010.499824. PMID: 22214443.

The fact that the woman described in the Bible suffered from strong blood flow already suggests a strong oestrogen effect (oestrogen dominance). One can well imagine that coupled with erotic fantasies, the mere touch of Jesus' garment could lead to a release of oxytocin and thus trigger strong—even haemorrhage stopping—uterine contractions. Interestingly, the Bible even describes that at the very moment she touched the garment, **she "felt" something in her womb** (Mark 5:29), which could be interpreted as violent uterine contractions.

Causes of Increased Oxytocin Release

- Birth (labour)
- Skin contact, (fur contact in animals), stroking, fondling, kissing
- Cognitive processes (erotic fantasies)
- Stimulation of the nipples
- Sexual intercourse, orgasm
- Rhythm and dance lead to oxytocin release
- Dates are eaten by Muslim women before birth, Oxytocin release.

1.22 Jesus Feeds the Five Thousand (The Miracle of Bread)

1.22.1 Original Text (Luke 9:10–17; Mark 6:30–44; Matthew 14:13–21; John 6:1–15)

Jesus Feeds the Five Thousand (Luke 9:10–17): 10 On their return, the apostles told him all that they had done. And he took them and withdrew apart to a town called Bethsaida. 11 When the crowds learned it, they followed him, and he welcomed them and spoke to them of the kingdom of God and cured those who had need of healing. 12 Now the day began to wear away, and the twelve came and said to him, "Send the crowd away to go into the surrounding villages and countryside to find lodging and get provisions, for we are here in a desolate place." 13 But he said to them, "You give them something to eat." They said, "We have no more than five loaves and two fish—unless we are to go and buy food for all these people." 14 For there were about five thousand men. And he said to his disciples, "**Have them sit down in groups of about fifty each.**" 15 And they did so, and had them all sit down. 16 And taking the five loaves and the two fish, he looked up to heaven and said a blessing over them. Then he broke the loaves and gave them to the disciples to set before the crowd. 17 And they all ate and were satisfied. And what was left over was picked up, twelve baskets of broken pieces.

Jesus Feeds the Five Thousand (Mark 6:30–44): 30 The apostles returned to Jesus and told him all that they had done and taught. 31 And he said to them, "Come away by yourselves to a desolate place and rest a while." For many were coming and going, and they had no leisure even to eat. 32 And they went away in the boat to a desolate place by themselves. 33 Now many saw them going and recognized them, and they ran there on foot from all the towns and got there ahead of them. 34 When he went ashore he saw a great crowd, and he had compassion on them, because they were like sheep without a shepherd. And he began to teach them many things. 35 And when it grew late, his disciples came to him and said, "This is a desolate place, and the hour is now late. 36 Send them away to go into the surrounding countryside and villages and buy themselves something to eat." 37 But he answered them, "You give them something to eat." And they said to him, "Shall we go and buy two hundred denarii[6] worth of bread and give it to them to eat?" 38 And he said to them, "How many loaves do you have? Go and see." And when they had found out, they said, "Five, and two fish." 39 Then he commanded them all to sit down in groups on the green grass. 40 So they sat down in groups, by hundreds and by fifties. 41 And taking the five loaves and the two fish, he looked up to heaven and said a blessing and broke the loaves and gave them to the disciples to set before the people. And he divided the two fish among them all. 42 And they all ate and were satisfied. 43 And they took up twelve baskets full of broken pieces and of the fish. 44 And those who ate the loaves were five thousand men.

Jesus Feeds the Five Thousand (Matthew 14:13–21): 13 Now when Jesus heard this, he withdrew from there in a boat to a desolate place by himself. But when the crowds heard it, they followed him on foot from the towns. 14 When he went ashore he saw a great crowd, and he had compassion on them and healed their sick. 15 Now when it was evening, the disciples came to him and said, "This is a desolate place, and the day is now over; send the crowds away to go into the villages and buy food for themselves." 16 But Jesus said, "They need not go away; you give them something to eat." 17 They said to him, "We have only five loaves here and two fish." 18 And he said, "Bring them here to me." 19 Then he ordered the crowds to sit down on the grass, and taking the five loaves and the two fish, he looked up to heaven and said a blessing. Then he broke the loaves and gave them to the disciples, and the disciples gave them to the crowds. 20 And they all ate and were satisfied. And they took up twelve baskets full of the broken pieces left over. 21 And those who ate were about five thousand men, besides women and children.

Jesus Feeds the Five Thousand (John 6:1–15): 1 After this Jesus went away to the other side of the Sea of Galilee, which is the Sea of Tiberias. 2 And a large crowd was following him, because they saw the signs that he was doing on the sick. 3 Jesus went up on the mountain, and there he sat down with his disciples. 4 Now the Passover, the feast of the Jews, was at hand. 5 Lifting up his eyes, then, and seeing that a large crowd was coming toward him, Jesus said to Philip, "Where are we to buy bread, so that these people may eat?" 6 He said this to test him, for he himself knew what he would do. 7 Philip answered him, "Two hundred denarii[1] worth of bread would not be enough for each of them to get a little." 8 One of his disciples, Andrew, Simon Peter's brother, said to him, 9 "There is a boy here who has five barley loaves and two fish, but what are they for so many?" 10 Jesus said, "Have the people sit down." Now there was much grass in the place. So the men sat down, about five thousand in number. 11 Jesus then took the loaves, and when he had given thanks, he distributed them to those who were seated. So also the fish, as much as they wanted. 12 And when they had eaten their fill, he told his disciples, "Gather up the leftover fragments, that nothing may be lost." 13 So they gathered them up and filled twelve baskets with fragments from the five barley loaves left by those who had eaten. 14 When the people saw the sign that he had done, they said, "This is indeed the Prophet who is to come into the world!" 15 Perceiving then that they were about to come and take him by force to make him king, Jesus withdrew again to the mountain by himself.

1.22.2 Description and Interpretation

After Jesus healed many people, more and more people followed him. Actually, he wanted to retire with his disciples and asked his disciples to take him by boat to the other side of the Sea of Galilee. However, the crowd found out about this plan and was already at the said place before Jesus and his disciples. About 5000 people were already waiting for him. So Jesus preached to them.

When evening came, his disciples told him to send the people home because they did not have enough bread with them, nor enough money to buy food for all 5000 people. Jesus asked his disciples how much food they had. They answered him: about 5 loaves and 2 fishes, which of course was far too little for all the listeners.

Jesus then told his disciples to ask the listeners to sit down on the grass and divide into groups of about 50 people. After the groups had formed, he went and got a little boy who was carrying 5 loaves and 2 fish. He said a prayer of thanksgiving, blessed and broke the loaves and fishes and distributed them. He told his disciples to distribute the loaves and fishes to all the listeners. Which they did. All 5000 listeners ate and were filled. In fact, there was so much food left over that the disciples were able to collect 12 baskets of leftovers. At least this is the story of the miraculous multiplication of the loaves.

On the one hand, Jesus and his disciples were exhausted after the miraculous healings and wanted to find a quiet place. On the other hand, more and more people followed the itinerant preacher. That might have been right for Jesus insofar as he could bring his views closer to many people at once. He talked to them in a friendly manner and explained the kingdom of God to them until evening finally came. As the day was running out, the disciples wanted to send the listeners away, especially since they feared supply problems. The audience had already grown to about 5,000 people, and they did not have nearly enough provisions to feed so many.

John's Gospel tells us that the **Passover was just around the corner** (John 6:4), a time when the Jews would normally set out on pilgrimage to Jerusalem to celebrate the Passover. Something similar still happens today with Muslims who go on the Hajj to make the pilgrimage to Mecca. Jesus knew this and could assume that the people who followed him had enough travel provisions with them. **No one would set out on a pilgrimage without taking enough provisions with them**.

Jesus recognized the situation, namely that there would be enough provisions if he managed to divide the available provisions equally among the 5000 listeners. Apparently, however, no one was willing to share their precious provisions. One can assume that everyone was afraid of not having enough left for himself if he started to divide his provisions. And now Jesus' social intelligence comes into play: he tells his disciples to divide the crowd into small groups and have them sit down on the grass. When you divide people into **small groups**, a group dynamic spontaneously develops. In small groups (the Bible says 50 persons) people's social behaviour follows very different rules compared with those in a mass of 5000 Genetically anchored, behaviours such as sharing food (**food sharing**) can thus be activated.[144] In addition, by asking people to sit down on the grass and make themselves comfortable,

[144] Barragan RC, Brooks R, Meltzoff AN. Altruistic food sharing behavior by human infants after a hunger manipulation. Sci Rep. 2020 Feb 4;10(1):1785. doi: https://doi.org/10.1038/s41598-020-58645-9. PMID: 32019998; PMCID: PMC7000707.

he created a pleasant social atmosphere. The time pressure was gone, the tension of expectation was released, and people could sit down in peace and chat with one another, thus **establishing social contacts**.

Nowadays, in a city with thousands of people flocking to the subway, such social behaviour would not even be possible. You can't exchange a few friendly words with everyone, and if you tried to do so, it would come across rather peculiar or even too much in-your-face. Due to the stimulus overload in cities, where no "normal contacts" can be made at all, social behaviour changes permanently. This phenomenon is also called "urban overload" by social psychologists and causes people's behaviour to become self-focused.[145] In the mass, people think mainly of themselves. Conversely, this self-focus can be changed quickly by splitting people up into small "manageable" groups, in which it becomes possible again to maintain social contacts and "care" for one another. But there is something else: If now in such a group a single person begins to share, the others also feel "obliged" to share. The more people begin to share, the stronger the peer pressure becomes, until finally everyone shares.[146] The whole effect of sharing is observed by the group members. This leads to another effect that social psychologists call "evaluation anxiety". Behavioural changes occur that reinforce social behaviour ("social facilitation")[147] and attenuate antisocial behaviour ("social loafing").[148] By splitting into small groups of 50 members, Jesus created the ideal conditions for helping behaviour.

Perhaps the proximity of Passover was also a factor in willingness to share bread and give up the left-overs just before the time when only unleavened bread (matzot) could be eaten.

Jesus was a fantastic psychologist, and adds an action to it by publicly showing all the people how a little boy is willing to give away and share his 5 loaves and 2 fish. **To reinforce this, he breaks the loaves and shares the fishes again publicly**. In doing so, he gives the sign that those camped in groups should do the same. In social psychology, one would call this today the creation of a "group rule".[149] To give this rule additional "divine" authority, he said a prayer of thanks to God, "blessed and broke it". Whoever stopped playing this game could be sure to be quickly excluded

---

145 "The experience of living in cities: A psychological analysis. - PsycNET." APA PsycNET, 10 Nov. 2021, https://doi.org/10.1037/10042-011.

146 Shteynberg G. Shared Attention. Perspect Psychol Sci. 2015 Sep;10(5):579–90. doi: https://doi.org/10.1177/1745691615589104. PMID: 26385997.

147 Herman CP. The social facilitation of eating. A review. Appetite. 2015 Mar;86:61–73. doi: https://doi.org/10.1016/j.appet.2014.09.016. Epub 2014 Sep 26. PMID: 25265153.

148 Hoeksema-van Orden CY, Gaillard AW, Buunk BP. Social loafing under fatigue. J Pers Soc Psychol. 1998 Nov;75(5):1179–90. doi: https://doi.org/10.1037//0022-3514.75.5.1179. PMID: 9866183.

149 Feldhege, Franz-Josef and Günter Krauthan. "Übungsheft für Klienten: Arbeitsunterlagen zum Verhaltenstrainingsprogramm zum Aufbau sozialer Kompetenz (VTP)." Allgemeine Gruppenregeln. Springer, 1979, pp. 4–5. doi: https://doi.org/10.1007/978-3-642-81312-2_1.

from his group.[150] Conversely, all with group-conforming behaviour could expect to receive social recognition.

As an itinerant preacher, Jesus knew the impact he had on the population, and in this situation he could assume that the majority of people would follow his example and unpack and share their provisions. Those who did not want to join in were very likely to be subjected to such high social pressure within their "group" that they were virtually forced to join in. So **the "miracle" was not that the bread and fish began to multiply, but that people began to share**. How abundantly supplied the people were with provisions could be seen from the fact that the apostles were still able to collect many baskets of leftover food.

Abstract: By forming small groups, a dynamic group behaviour is created that leads thousands of people to bring out the provisions they brought themselves and share them with the others. This allowed 5,000 people to be miraculously satiated.

1.23 Jesus Walks on the Water

1.23.1 Original Text (Mark 6:45–52; Matthew 14:22–33; John 6:16–21)

Jesus Walks on the Water (Mark 6:45–52): 45 Immediately he made his disciples get into the boat and go before him to the other side, to Bethsaida, while he dismissed the crowd. 46 And after he had taken leave of them, he went up on the mountain to pray. 47 And when evening came, the boat was out on the sea, and he was alone on the land. 48 And he saw that they were making headway painfully, for the wind was against them. And about the fourth watch of the night he came to them, walking on the sea. He meant to pass by them, 49 but when they saw him walking on the sea they thought it was a ghost, and cried out, 50 for they all saw him and were terrified. But immediately he spoke to them and said, "Take heart; it is I. Do not be afraid." 51 And he got into the boat with them, and the wind ceased. And they were utterly astounded, 52 for they did not understand about the loaves, but their hearts were hardened.

Jesus Walks on the Water (Matthew 14:22–33): 22 Immediately he made the disciples get into the boat and go before him to the other side, while he dismissed the crowds. 23 And after he had dismissed the crowds, he went up on the mountain by himself to pray. When evening came, he was there alone, 24 but the boat by this time was a long way from the land, beaten by the waves, for the wind was against them. 25 And in the fourth watch of the night he came to them, walking on the sea. 26 But when the disciples saw him walking on the sea, they were terrified, and said, "It is a ghost!" and they cried out in fear. 27 But immediately Jesus spoke to them, saying, "Take heart; it is I. Do not be afraid." 28 And Peter answered him, "Lord, if it is you, command me to come to you on the water." 29 He said, "Come." So Peter got out of the boat and walked on the water and came to Jesus. 30 But when he saw the wind, he was afraid, and beginning to sink he cried out, "Lord, save me." 31 Jesus immediately reached out his hand and took hold of him, saying to him, "O you of little faith,

[150] Ditrich, Lara and Kai Sassenberg. "Einer ohne alle oder alle ohne Einen? Eine sozialpsychologische Perspektive auf Ausschluss und Austritt aus Gruppen." Zeitschrift für Kulturwissenschaften, vol. 10, no. 2, 1 Nov. 2016, pp. 23–36. doi: https://doi.org/10.14361/zfk-2016-0203.

why did you doubt?" 32 And when they got into the boat, the wind ceased. 33 And those in the boat worshipped him, saying, "Truly you are the Son of God."

Jesus Walks on Water (John 6:16–2): 16 When evening came, his disciples went down to the sea, 17 got into a boat, and started across the sea to Capernaum. It was now dark, and Jesus had not yet come to them. 18 The sea became rough because a strong wind was blowing. 19 When they had rowed about three or four miles, they saw Jesus walking on the sea and coming near the boat, and they were frightened. 20 But he said to them, "It is I; do not be afraid." 21 Then they were glad to take him into the boat, and immediately the boat was at the land to which they were going.

1.23.2 Description and Interpretation

After the miraculous multiplication of bread and fish, in which about 5000 people were fed, the disciples wanted to return to Capernaum via the Sea of Galilee. Jesus asked his disciples to go ahead alone. Meantime, he was going to send the people home. The boat with the disciples was already several stadia (about 5–6 km) from the shore when a sudden storm came up and the boat was tossed back and forth. The disciples in the boat became very frightened. Suddenly, one of the disciples saw a figure coming across the lake to their boat. The others also saw the figure and thought it was a ghost. They cried out in fear, but the figure tried to calm them down and said to them, "do not be afraid", trust, it is me. Then they recognized Jesus in the figure. Peter tried to cross the water to meet him. He sank and cried out to Jesus, "Lord, save me". Jesus reached out his hand and took hold of him, scolding Peter for having so little faith in him. But by the time they got him into the boat, they were already on the safe shore they had originally intended to reach.

The area where the apostles were going to cross the lake is known for sudden thermal winds that can be very strong. These strong winds still exist today, which is why it is advertised on the Internet as "Europe's most popular region for wind surfers".[151] The Bible says that a sudden storm arose and the disciples who were in the boat were really afraid. Fear is known to be a common trigger for hallucinations.[152] It is likely that the accompanying hyperventilation leads to electrolyte shifts, resulting in hallucinatory perceptual disturbances. In the context of such perceptual disturbances, it is easy to imagine that, for example, a log floating in the water is suddenly seen as a "saving saviour". **A classical case for an illusion or illusionary misperception.**[153]

The question arises, how it happened that apparently all the travellers in the boat could have hallucinations or illusory misperceptions and see Jesus walking on

[151] "Israel: See Genetareth." Www.surf-magazin, 5 Oct. 2018, www.surf-magazin.de/reisen/naher_osten/israel-see-genetareth.

[152] Ratcliffe M, Wilkinson S. How anxiety induces verbal hallucinations. Conscious Cogn. 2016 Jan;39:48–58. doi: https://doi.org/10.1016/j.concog.2015.11.009. Epub 2015 Dec 9. PMID: 26683229; PMCID: PMC4710580.

[153] Todorović D. What Are Visual Illusions? Perception. 2020 Nov;49(11):1128–1199. doi: https://doi.org/10.1177/0301006620962279. PMID: 33183136.

the water. This is where the miraculous fish multiplication comes in. About two days' walk from where Jesus preached, sea bream (Sarpa salpa), also known as "dream fish" because they contain a hallucinogen with LSD-like effects, are found in the Mediterranean Sea. The longer it takes to process the fish, the stronger the hallucinatory effect of this fish toxin becomes. Thus, a few hours after eating the fish, hallucinations and delirious states can occur, which can last for several hours.

Such fish poisonings, called "**ichthyoallyeinotoxism**" (ICD-10 T43), are also known in modern times[154] and usually affect groups of people who have shared such a meal. Exactly which toxin is involved is not yet known, but it has similar effects to the known fish toxins **ciguatoxin** and **maitotoxin.**[155] These toxins **have neurotoxic effects**, blocking voltage-dependent sodium channels of nerve cells.[156] Maitotoxin acts on calcium channels.[157] These compounds can lead to various neurological symptoms, including vivid hallucinations and altered perceptions. The toxins do not harm the fish, but **cause symptoms of illness similar to LSD intoxication in humans who eat these fish**. Heating does not destroy these toxins, which is why they continue to cause intoxication symptoms even after preparation. **Similar to the description of an LSD trip when people suddenly believe they can fly, Peter also believes he can walk on water and sinks**, reportedly because he didn't really believe in the power of Jesus. Similar incidents are described again and again today, when people who take drugs believing they can fly jump out of windows and crash. Just as then, also today, affected persons have the tendency to transform a "horror trip" into a "good experience".[158]

Probably, however, Jesus' apparition was not a real hallucination at all, but only an illusory misperception, meaning that some object—driftwood, for example—was floating on the water. This would also explain that Peter finally could cling to "Jesus" (respectively, i.e. the driftwood) and then did not drown after all. Fear together with

---

[154] de Haro L, Pommier P. Hallucinatory fish poisoning (ichthyoallyeinotoxism): two case reports from the Western Mediterranean and literature review. Clin Toxicol (Phila). 2006;44(2):185–8. doi: https://doi.org/10.1080/15563650500514590. PMID: 16615678.

[155] Bellassoued K, Van Pelt J, Elfeki A. Neurotoxicity in rats induced by the poisonous dreamfish (Sarpa salpa). Pharm Biol. 2015 Feb;53(2):286–95. doi: https://doi.org/10.3109/13880209.2014.916311. Epub 2014 Sep 22. PMID: 25243872.

[156] Inserra MC, Israel MR, Caldwell A, Castro J, Deuis JR, Harrington AM, Keramidas A, Garcia-Caraballo S, Maddern J, Erickson A, Grundy L, Rychkov GY, Zimmermann K, Lewis RJ, Brierley SM, Vetter I. Multiple sodium channel isoforms mediate the pathological effects of Pacific ciguatoxin-1. Sci Rep. 2017 Feb 22;7:42810. doi: https://doi.org/10.1038/srep42810. PMID: 28225079; PMCID: PMC5320492.

[157] Gusovsky F, Daly JW. Maitotoxin: a unique pharmacological tool for research on calcium-dependent mechanisms. Biochem Pharmacol. 1990 Jun 1;39(11):1633–9. doi: https://doi.org/10.1016/0006-2952(90)90105-t. PMID: 1971510.

[158] Gashi L, Sandberg S, Pedersen W. Making "bad trips" good: How users of psychedelics narratively transform challenging trips into valuable experiences. Int J Drug Policy. 2021 Jan;87:102997. doi: https://doi.org/10.1016/j.drugpo.2020.102997. Epub 2020 Oct 17. Erratum in: Int J Drug Policy. 2021 Jul;93:103183. PMID: 33080454.

hallucinogenic poisons from a spoiled fish meal seem to be reason enough to have such experiences, which are later rationalized in the form of a miraculous story.

Abstract: An explanation for the miracle of Jesus walking on the water would be the following: Fish poisoning with hallucinogenic fish toxin → ichthyoallyeinotoxism → illusory misperception or hallucination of a whole group that sees Jesus walking on the water. Fear and hyperventilation play a role only as triggers. **Nowadays, the diagnosis would be**: hallucination (ICD-10 T44) with "**ichthyoallyeinotoxism**" (ICD-10 T43) **triggered by anxiety**-induced hyperventilation (ICD-10 R45).

1.24 The Syro-Phoenician Woman's Faith (Remote Healing of the Daughter of a Foreigner)

1.24.1 Original Text (Mark 7:24–30; Matthew 15:21–28)

The Syro-Phoenician Woman's Faith (Mark 7:24–30): 24 And from there he arose and went away to the region of Tyre and Sidon. And he entered a house and did not want anyone to know, yet he could not be hidden. 25 But immediately a woman whose little daughter had an unclean spirit heard of him and came and fell down at his feet. 26 Now the woman was a Gentile, a Syro-Phoenician by birth. And she begged him to cast the demon out of her daughter. 27 And he said to her, "Let the children be fed first, for it is not right to take the children's bread and throw it to the dogs." 28 But she answered him, "Yes, Lord; yet even the dogs under the table eat the children's crumbs." 29 And he said to her, "For this statement you may go your way; the demon has left your daughter." 30 And she went home and found the child lying in bed and the demon gone.

The Faith of a Canaanite Woman (Matthew 15:21–28): 21 And Jesus went away from there and withdrew to the district of Tyre and Sidon. 22 And behold, a Canaanite woman from that region came out and was crying, "Have mercy on me, O Lord, Son of David; my daughter is severely oppressed by a demon." 23 But he did not answer her a word. And his disciples came and begged him, saying, "Send her away, for she is crying out after us." 24 He answered, "I was sent only to the lost sheep of the house of Israel." 25 But she came and knelt before him, saying, "Lord, help me." 26 And he answered, "It is not right to take the children's bread and throw it to the dogs." 27 She said, "Yes, Lord, yet even the dogs eat the crumbs that fall from their masters' table." 28 Then Jesus answered her, "O woman, great is your faith! Be it done for you as you desire." And her daughter was healed instantly.

1.24.2 Description and Interpretation

Jesus travels with his disciples to the region of Sidon and Tyre (Phoenicia). He finds a house there where he can stay, but wants to prevent his stay from becoming public knowledge. But again he does not succeed. A woman of Canaanite descent, born in this region, comes to him and asks: "Lord, have mercy on me! My daughter is possessed by a demon". But Jesus does not respond. After a while, the disciples urged him, "Send her away, she's been screaming after us all the time!" Then Jesus explained why he didn't pay attention to her, "I was sent only to the lost sheep of Israel".

But the woman does not give up. She falls on her knees before Jesus and pleads, "Lord, help me!". To find out how great her faith is, he alludes to the negative image the Jews had of foreign peoples he says, "It is not right to take the bread away from the children (meaning the Jews) and throw it to the little dogs (meaning Gentiles)". To this, the woman replied, "Yes, sir, but the little dogs also eat the crumbs that fall from their master's table". Then he realizes how strong the faith of this woman is, and he says: "Your faith is great. What you wish shall be done". And that's exactly what happened. Although her daughter was not around, she was healed. When the woman came home, she sees her daughter lying in bed, completely healthy and free from the demon.

Usually, this somewhat strange text is interpreted by theologians in such a way that first one's own children—meaning the Jews—are to be provided with bread. Only afterwards does one give the bread crumbs to the dogs, meaning thereby the Gentiles and heathens. The woman answers that, however, also the dogs (Gentiles) get something to eat from the bread crumbs. Whether this interpretation is correct or not, remains to be seen. Here it is shown that a pagan woman had a very strong faith in Jesus and his healing powers. It is also shown that [when there is] a strong faith, similar to the case of the Roman officer whose servant lay sick at home, healings are possible even from a distance, even in unbelievers and Gentiles. **The decisive factor is always the unshakeable *faith* in healing**. Jesus also does not claim that healing will occur, but always says "let it happen as you have imagined or as you have believed". This is the basic prerequisite for a self-fulfilling prophecy[159] or placebo effect by suggestion.

Unfortunately, nothing is written here about the "nature of the possession" and about accompanying symptoms, so that no further interpretation can be made. However, remote healing always has a lot to do with faith and placebo effects.

Objectively, the daughter may not have changed at all, but, under the influence of faith, the mother perceived her daughter as having been cured. Alternatively, it may be that the daughter was simply a normal, rebellious teenager. In that case, it is also possible that the daughter was so impressed by the mother's story about her encounter with the holy man that she became more obedient. It is also possible that, even before the mother's encounter with Jesus, the daughter was impressed with the extent of her mother's concern about her behaviour and changed her disobedient ways.

Abstract: Self-fulfilling prophecy.

[159] Glaser, Christian. "Risiko im Management: 100 Fehler, Irrtümer, Verzerrungen und wie man sie vermeidet." Selbsterfüllende Prophezeiung. Springer Gabler, 7 May. 2019, pp. 81–84. doi: https://doi.org/10.1007/978-3-658-25835-1_21.

1.25 Jesus Heals a Deaf Man (The Healing of the Deaf-Mute in Decapolis)

1.25.1 Original Text (Mark 7:31–37, Matthew 15:29–31)

Jesus Heals a Deaf Man (Mark 7:31–37): 31 Then he returned from the region of Tyre and went through Sidon to the Sea of Galilee, in the region of the Decapolis. 32 And they brought to him a man who was deaf and had a speech impediment, and they begged him to lay his hand on him. 33 And taking him aside from the crowd privately, he put his fingers into his ears, and after spitting touched his tongue. 34 And looking up to heaven, he sighed and said to him, "Ephphatha," that is, "Be opened." 35 And his ears were opened, his tongue was released, and he spoke plainly. 36 And Jesus[8] charged them to tell no one. But the more he charged them, the more zealously they proclaimed it. 37 And they were astonished beyond measure, saying, "He has done all things well. He even makes the deaf hear and the mute speak."

Jesus Heals Many (Matthew 15:29–31): 29 Jesus went on from there and walked beside the Sea of Galilee. And he went up on the mountain and sat down there. 30 And great crowds came to him, bringing with them the lame, the blind, the crippled, the mute, and many others, and they put them at his feet, and he healed them, 31 so that the crowd wondered, when they saw the mute speaking, the crippled healthy, the lame walking, and the blind seeing. And they glorified the God of Israel.

1.25.2 Description and Interpretation

Jesus came again to the Sea of Galilee in the region of Decapolis. Then the people brought to Jesus a man who was deaf and could ***hardly*** speak, and asked him to lay hands on him. Jesus took the deaf man aside, away from the crowd, and put his fingers in his ears. Then he touched the man's tongue with his saliva. He looked up to heaven and said, "open up". Immediately, the man could hear again and speak properly. As before, he forbade the man to tell anyone about it. But the more he forbade it, the more people told about his miracles and people marvelled at his ability to work miracles.

Everyone knows expressions such as "it makes me speechless". Expressions are always an indication that a pathophysiological process occurs frequently or is observed again and again. When a writer wants to express anxiety, he may describe a situation "as someone speaks with a shaky voice", etc. People who stutter worsen their speech when they are stressed. The voice very often reveals the stress level someone is in, as well as the current "mood". Jesus obviously sensed that the man involved was stressed. Therefore, he took him aside, away from all other people and bystanders. This was the prerequisite for a confidential and relaxed atmosphere.

In the present case **a stammering voice is mentioned,** in the Ebenfeld Bible this passage is translated as "**someone who spoke with difficulty**". Also in other translations **the person concerned was not mute, but could still talk, but just**

with difficulty. Dyslalia[160] (ICD F80.0) or stuttering[161] (ICD F98.5) would be the medical terms that could be applied here. In addition, there is the statement that the man was "deaf". He could not have been completely deaf from birth, otherwise he would not have been able to speak at all. In order to learn language, a certain hearing ability must be present. **And he could speak, he just could not speak "fluently"**. So if he was only temporarily deaf, of course **psychogenic deafness**[162] is a possibility (ICD F44.6; synonyms for psychogenic deafness are hysterical deafness, emotional deafness or functional deafness). In this form of deafness, the hearing organ is, objectively speaking, intact. That is, when measuring hearing with modern methods which do not require cooperation of the subject, "normal" results can be obtained. Subjectively, however, the person concerned hears nothing. The sound arrives in the brain, but is not further processed there. The most **frequent cause of this type of psychogenic deafness is mental stress or psychological trauma**. After World Wars 1 and 2, this disorder was increasingly described. In a paper by Kiefer published in 2005, six such patients were described and treated. In five out of six patients, a complete subjective production of hearing could be achieved by **psychosuggestive methods** alone.[163]

Anyone who knows a stutterer knows that such speech disorders worsen in situations of excitement and improve at rest. Anyone who works with people suffering from mental distress knows that by creating calm or by reassuring them, symptoms can be improved. Jesus did just that in this case. He "took the man aside" i.e. he shielded him from the environment and thus created a calm atmosphere which must have been essential for the healing success. By the unusual measure of touching a stranger with his own saliva, inserting a finger into the ear and a (theatrical) sigh to the sky and the subsequent suggestive command "be opened" he undoubtedly performed a suggestive manipulation or in modern terms a psychosuggestive therapy. Suggestive manipulation is also known by the term placebo effect. Also interesting is that even today, saliva is associated with magic. Some people still simulate spitting on the dice when playing dice, promising themselves good luck. Likewise, even today during initiation rites of some yoga directions (Surat-Shabd Yoga), the guru puts his finger in the ear of the adept to be accepted, with the aim of opening the "inner" ear of the adept. Apparently, man had and still has a certain inclination to esoteric rituals and likes to be manipulated with them.

Abstract: Dyslalia (ICD F80.0) or stuttering (ICD F98.5) and intermittent psychogenic deafness (ICD F44.6). Cure by psychosuggestive therapy.

---

160 Takaoka K, Shibata K. [Speech articulation disorder (dyslalia)]. Ryoikibetsu Shokogun Shirizu. 2003;(39):483–6. Japanese. PMID: 14503320.

161 Prasse JE, Kikano GE. Stuttering: an overview. Am Fam Physician. 2008 May 1;77(9):1271–6. PMID: 18540491.

162 Ban JH, Jin SM. A clinical analysis of psychogenic sudden deafness. Otolaryngol Head Neck Surg. 2006 Jun;134(6):970–4. doi: https://doi.org/10.1016/j.otohns.2005.11.045. PMID: 16730540.

163 J. Kiefer 1, W. Arnold 1: Ein Verfahren zur Therapie der akuten, psychogenen Hörstörung; HNO-Informationen (Kongressabstracts) 2005; 84–444. https://doi.org/10.1055/s-2005-869192.

1.26 Jesus Heals a Blind Man at Bethsaida (The Healing of the Blind Man of Bethsaida)

1.26.1 Original Text (Mark 8:22–26)

Jesus Heals a Blind Man at Bethsaida (Mark 8:22–26): 22 And they came to Bethsaida. And some people brought to him a blind man and begged him to touch him. 23 And he took the blind man by the hand and led him out of the village, and when he had spit on his eyes and laid his hands on him, he asked him, "Do you see anything?" 24 And he looked up and said, "I see people, but they look like trees, walking." 25 Then Jesus[3] laid his hands on his eyes again; and he opened his eyes, his sight was restored, and he saw everything clearly. 26 And he sent him to his home, saying, "Do not even enter the village."

1.26.2 Description and Interpretation

When Jesus and his disciples came to Bethsaida, the people brought a blind man to him so that he might touch him and heal him. Jesus led the blind man out of the village. There he put saliva on the blind man's eyes and asked him if he could see anything. The blind man answered, "**I see people, but they look like trees, walking**". Jesus then placed his hands on the blind man's eyes once again. After that, the blind man could see "normally" again. Jesus sent him home again, but did instruct him not to go back to the village.

Jesus obviously knew that he would have better success if he did not perform his treatments in front of the gathered crowd. On the one hand, this created a more trusting atmosphere, which also promised better "healing results". On the other hand, he was also better protected, if the healing should fail. In the whole Bible only the successful healings are recorded, but unsuccessful healing attempts, which probably also existed, are never mentioned. If he was alone in a healing attempt and experienced failure, this could rather be swept under the carpet.

If a person says a sentence like "I see the people, because I see them walking around like trees", then that makes us think first of all perception disturbances. Hearing the phrase: "walking around like trees", one is most likely to think of **illusory misperception** or **pseudohallucination**,[164] because there is an external stimulus (namely people), but they are misinterpreted (namely trees) and the person concerned recognizes the impossibility of what is seen. Exactly this phenomenon exists in blind people and is called **Charles Bonnet Syndrome** (CBS).[165] In this case, isolated visual hallucinations occur in blind or poorly sighted patients, but who do not have a psychiatric illness. It occurs primarily in people who are gradually losing their

---

[164] DocCheck Medical Services GmbH. "Pseudohalluzination - DocCheck Flexikon." DocCheck Flexikon, 4 Nov. 2021, flexikon.doccheck.com/de/Pseudohalluzination.

[165] Hamedani AG, Pelak VS. The Charles Bonnet Syndrome: a Systematic Review of Diagnostic Criteria. Curr Treat Options Neurol. 2019 Jul 25;21(9):41. doi: https://doi.org/10.1007/s11940-019-0582-1. Erratum in: Curr Treat Options Neurol. 2019 Oct 4;21(10):52. PMID: 31342218.

vision. Triggering conditions include cataracts,[166] diabetic retinopathy,[167] macular degeneration,[168] and other eye diseases such as haemorrhages, tumours, and cerebral infarcts. Migraines or drugs can also cause similar symptoms.[169] It is important that the affected person recognizes the "falseness" of the hallucinations, which is the case in the present description: he does not say "I see people", but "I see them walking around like trees". There is no better way to describe a pseudohallucination, because unlike real hallucinations, the sufferer recognizes that his vision cannot be real. When the pseudo-hallucinations are over, the affected person sees as before, mostly badly, but they perceive it as "normal". In the case of migraine-induced Charles Bonnet syndrome (status migrainosus), full visual acuity may be restored.

The exact cause of Charles Bonnet Syndrome (CBS) is still not precisely known, but psychosocial factors are likely to play an important role.[170] Stimulus deficiency, social isolation and cognitive deficits are likely to contribute to the development of CBS.[171] Sufferers, are not only stressed by the complex hallucinatory experiences, but are also afraid of going crazy or being seen as crazy if they talk about it. This fear is all the more pronounced, especially since those affected, mostly old people, do indeed have insight that these are hallucinations and not actual experiences. Loneliness is in any case a trigger for hallucinations in the context of a CBS. This could also be seen during the lock-downs in the context of the Covid-19 pandemic. During this time, the incidence of CBS increased significantly.[172] Social isolation and thus hallucinations can be broken through attention. Jesus of Nazareth repeatedly distinguished himself

---

[166] Smith CS, Nichols J, Riaz KM. Remission of Charles Bonnet syndrome after cataract extraction. Can J Ophthalmol. 2018 Dec;53(6):e221–e222. doi: https://doi.org/10.1016/j.jcjo.2018.01.036. Epub 2018 Apr 2. PMID: 30502996.

[167] Carvalho NP, Fasanya O, McNally S. Charles Bonnet syndrome in a young adult with diabetic retinopathy. Br J Hosp Med (Lond). 2021 Aug 2;82(8):1–2. doi: https://doi.org/10.12968/hmed.2021.0012. Epub 2021 Aug 7. PMID: 34431352.

[168] Niazi S, Krogh Nielsen M, Singh A, Sørensen TL, Subhi Y. Prevalence of Charles Bonnet syndrome in patients with age-related macular degeneration: systematic review and meta-analysis. Acta Ophthalmol. 2020 Mar;98(2):121–131. doi: https://doi.org/10.1111/aos.14287. Epub 2019 Oct 26. PMID: 31654492.

[169] Casas J, Baños JE, Guardiola E. Las alucinaciones visuales en la obra de Oliver Sacks [Visual hallucinations in the works of Oliver Sacks]. Rev Neurol. 2020 Jan 16;70(2):67–71. Spanish. doi: https://doi.org/10.33588/rn.7002.2019267. PMID: 31930472.

[170] Jones L, Ditzel-Finn L, Enoch J, Moosajee M. An overview of psychological and social factors in Charles Bonnet syndrome. Ther Adv Ophthalmol. 2021 Jul 30;13:25158414211034715. doi: https://doi.org/10.1177/25158414211034715. PMID: 34377938; PMCID: PMC8330457.

[171] Menon GJ, Rahman I, Menon SJ, Dutton GN. Complex visual hallucinations in the visually impaired: the Charles Bonnet Syndrome. Surv Ophthalmol. 2003 Jan–Feb;48(1):58–72. doi: https://doi.org/10.1016/s0039-6257(02)00414-9. PMID: 12559327.

[172] Jones L, Ditzel-Finn L, Potts J, Moosajee M. Exacerbation of visual hallucinations in Charles Bonnet syndrome due to the social implications of COVID-19. BMJ Open Ophthalmol. 2021 Feb 11;6(1):e000670. doi: https://doi.org/10.1136/bmjophth-2020-000670. PMID: 33628948; PMCID: PMC7880118.

by a special empathy. So one can well imagine that just by loving attention,[173] hallucination in the context of a CBS were interrupted and thus "cured".

Jesus, of course, could not have known Charles Bonnet Syndrome, nor could he have known the difference between real hallucination and pseudohallucination. But it is interesting that symptoms were described thousands of years ago that we are only able to explain today.

Abstract: **Pseudohallucinations** in the context of a **Charles Bonnet syndrome** (ICD-10: F06.0).

1.27 Jesus Heals a Boy with an Unclean Spirit (The Healing of the Moonstruck Boy, the Unsuccessful Disciples)

1.27.1 Original Text (Luke 9:37–43; Mark 9:14–29)

Jesus Heals a Boy with an Unclean Spirit (Luke 9:37–43): 37 On the next day, when they had come down from the mountain, a great crowd met him. 38 And behold, a man from the crowd cried out, "Teacher, I beg you to look at my son, for he is my only child. 39 And behold, a spirit seizes him, and he suddenly cries out. It convulses him so that he foams at the mouth, and shatters him, and will hardly leave him. 40 And I begged your disciples to cast it out, but they could not." 41 Jesus answered, "O faithless and twisted generation, how long am I to be with you and bear with you? Bring your son here." 42 While he was coming, the demon threw him to the ground and convulsed him. But Jesus rebuked the unclean spirit and healed the boy, and gave him back to his father.

Jesus Heals a Boy with an Unclean Spirit (Mark 9:14–29): 14 And when they came to the disciples, they saw a great crowd around them, and scribes arguing with them. 15 And immediately all the crowd, when they saw him, were greatly amazed and ran up to him and greeted him. 16 And he asked them, "What are you arguing about with them?" 17 And someone from the crowd answered him, "Teacher, I brought my son to you, for he has a spirit that makes him mute. 18 And whenever it seizes him, it throws him down, and he foams and grinds his teeth and becomes rigid. So I asked your disciples to cast it out, and they were not able." 19 And he answered them, "O faithless generation, how long am I to be with you? How long am I to bear with you? Bring him to me." 20 And they brought the boy to him. And when the spirit saw him, immediately it convulsed the boy, and he fell on the ground and rolled about, foaming at the mouth. 21 And Jesus asked his father, "How long has this been happening to him?" And he said, "From childhood. 22 And it has often cast him into fire and into water, to destroy him. But if you can do anything, have compassion on us and help us." 23 And Jesus said to him, "'If you can'! All things are possible for one who believes." 24 Immediately, the father of the child cried out and said, "I believe; help my unbelief!" 25 And when Jesus saw that a crowd came running together, he rebuked the unclean spirit, saying to it, "You mute and deaf spirit, I command you, come out of him and never enter him again." 26 And after crying out and convulsing him terribly, it came out,

---

[173] Ophthalmol. 2003 Jan–Feb;48(1):58–72. doi: https://doi.org/10.1016/s0039-6257(02)00414-9. PMID: 12559327. Jones L, Ditzel-Finn L, Potts J, Moosajee M. Exacerbation of visual hallucinations in Charles Bonnet syndrome due to the social implications of COVID-19. BMJ Open Ophthalmol. 2021 Feb 11;6(1):e000670. doi: https://doi.org/10.1136/bmjophth-2020-000670. PMID: 33628948; PMCID: PMC7880118.

and the boy was like a corpse, so that most of them said, "He is dead." 27 But Jesus took him by the hand and lifted him up, and he arose. 28 And when he had entered the house, his disciples asked him privately, "Why could we not cast it out?" 29 And he said to them, "This kind cannot be driven out by anything but prayer."

Jesus Heals a Boy with a Demon (Matthew 17:14–21): 14 And when they came to the crowd, a man came up to him and, kneeling before him, 15 said, "Lord, have mercy on my son, for he has seizures and he suffers terribly. For often he falls into the fire, and often into the water. 16 And I brought him to your disciples, and they could not heal him." 17 And Jesus answered, "O faithless and twisted generation, how long am I to be with you? How long am I to bear with you? Bring him here to me." 18 And Jesus rebuked the demon, and it came out of him, and the boy was healed instantly. 19 Then the disciples came to Jesus privately and said, "Why could we not cast it out?" 20 He said to them, "Because of your little faith. For truly, I say to you, if you have faith like a grain of mustard seed, you will say to this mountain, 'Move from here to there,' and it will move, and nothing will be impossible for you."

1.27.2 Description and Interpretation

When Jesus came down from a mountain with Peter, James and John, they saw a large crowd standing around the other disciples. Among them were scribes who were arguing with the disciples. When the crowd spotted Jesus, they ran to him. Jesus asked what they were arguing about. A man knelt down in front of Jesus and told him that he had a son who was possessed by an evil spirit. The demon kept throwing his son to the ground and then the boy foamed at the mouth, gnashed his teeth and became completely rigid (Mark 9:18). "I have already asked your disciples to cast out the evil spirit, but they did not succeed," he continued. Please Lord help my son.

Jesus was apparently annoyed that his disciples were not able to heal the boy, and thought they were of too little faith to be able to heal successfully. He then asked the boy's father how long he had had this evil spirit. The father answered that he had been possessed since childhood, and that the demon kept trying to kill him by throwing him into the fire or water (Mark 9:22). Jesus said to bring the boy to him. They fetched the boy and he *ran* to Jesus. As soon as he arrived at Jesus, the evil spirit attacked him again. The boy fell to the ground, rolled back and forth, convulsed and foamed at the mouth. Jesus ordered the evil spirit to leave the boy and never return. Then the demon left the boy with a shout. After that, the boy lay on the ground as if dead, so that people thought he had died. But Jesus took him by the hand, raised him up, and the boy arose.

Here **a case of infantile epilepsy** is described very beautifully.[174] Again and again the boy falls to the ground. In former times therefore it was also called the "**falling sickness**".[175] Further symptoms are described: how the child lying on the ground convulsed, had foam at the mouth, screamed loudly and bit himself in the tongue and/or gnashed his teeth. Afterwards, he lay on the floor "as if dead", so that people

[174] Park JT, Shahid AM, Jammoul A. Common pediatric epilepsy syndromes. Pediatr Ann. 2015 Feb;44(2):e30–5. doi: https://doi.org/10.3928/00904481-20150203-09. PMID: 25658216.

[175] "Fallsucht – Mittelalter-Lexikon." 16 Oct. 2021, www.mittelalter-lexikon.de/wiki/Fallsucht.

thought he had died. A good description for a so-called "**postictal stupor**".[176] Jesus asks the father how long he has had these conditions, and gets the answer that these complaints have existed since childhood.

Childhood epilepsies usually follow a very severe course, frequently with multiple epileptic seizures occurring daily. The cause of childhood epilepsies is usually found to be congenital metabolic disorders. One of them is the so-called **GLUT-1 transporter defect**, which is caused **by a mutation of the SLC2A1 gene**.[177] In this case, glucose (blood sugar) can no longer be adequately transported from the bloodstream into the brain. This leads to a so-called **hypoglycorrhachia**,[178] a **decrease of glucose in the cerebrospinal fluid**, while the blood glucose level remains normal. Even today, diagnosis is not easy because blood glucose is normal and glucose determinations in cerebrospinal fluid (CSF) are not routinely performed. Typically, **affected individuals show neurohypoglycaemic symptoms such as movement disorders (dyskinesias) and epileptic seizures**. Seizures are **triggered by physical exertion**, because here the blood sugar is increasingly consumed by the muscles and the brain enters an energy deficit with the consequence of an epileptic seizure. So if the child was brought "quickly" to Jesus and *had to run there* and then immediately suffered another seizure once there, this is another sign of such a "**Paroxysmal exercise-induced epilepsy**".[179] In any case, symptoms such as foaming at the mouth, convulsions and gnashing teeth are a sure sign of a so-called "**Grand Mal seizure**",[180] which is also consistent with the subsequent "**postictal stupor**".[181] (He lay there as if dead, and everyone said he died). A grand mal seizure, as it is written in the medical text book.

Apparently, the disciples had already tried to "cast out the evil spirit" before Jesus arrived, but without success. Jesus managed to heal the boy, and here **interesting translation variations** come into play, which are essential for the explanation of the "miracle healing"! While in all German Bible translations it is written in Mark

---

[176] Subota A, Khan S, Josephson CB, Manji S, Lukmanji S, Roach P, Wiebe S, Buchhalter J, Federico P, Teskey GC, Lorenzetti DL, Jetté N. Signs and symptoms of the postictal period in epilepsy: A systematic review and meta-analysis. Epilepsy Behav. 2019 May;94:243–251. doi: https://doi.org/10.1016/j.yebeh.2019.03.014. Epub 2019 Apr 9. PMID: 30978637.

[177] Wang D, Pascual JM, De Vivo D. Glucose Transporter Type 1 Deficiency Syndrome. 2002 Jul 30 [updated 2018 Mar 1]. In: Adam MP, Ardinger HH, Pagon RA, Wallace SE, Bean LJH, Mirzaa G, Amemiya A, editors. GeneReviews® [Internet]. Seattle (WA): University of Washington, Seattle; 1993–2021. PMID: 20301603.

[178] Chow E, Troy SB. The differential diagnosis of hypoglycorrhachia in adult patients. Am J Med Sci. 2014 Sep;348(3):186–90. doi: https://doi.org/10.1097/MAJ.0000000000000217. PMID: 24326618; PMCID: PMC4065645.

[179] Mongin M, Mezouar N, Dodet P, Vidailhet M, Roze E. Paroxysmal Exercise-induced Dyskinesias Caused by GLUT1 Deficiency Syndrome. Tremor Other Hyperkinet Mov (NY). 2016 Mar 4;6:371. doi: https://doi.org/10.7916/D89W0F96. PMID: 27351150; PMCID: PMC4790204.

[180] Jacobs, Julia. "Epilepsie: Tipps für Ersthelfer – Keine Gewalt bei Krampfanfall." ergopraxis, vol. 7, no. 02, Feb. 2014, pp. 28–29. doi: https://doi.org/10.1055/s-0034-1370374.

[181] Pottkämper JCM, Hofmeijer J, van Waarde JA, van Putten MJAM. The postictal state—What do we know? Epilepsia. 2020 Jun;61(6):1045–1061. doi: https://doi.org/10.1111/epi.16519. Epub 2020 May 12. PMID: 32396219; PMCID: PMC7317965.

9:28 "this kind can be cast out only by prayer", in the other translations (Latin, Italian, English) it is written that the healing can be achieved only by prayer and by *fasting*. The word "fasting", was suppressed in some **translations**. Apparently, the word "fasting" was not considered important by the translators. But it is precisely the "fasting" that is the key to the healing of infantile epilepsies, which develop on the basis of a GLUT-1 defect. If glucose cannot be adequately pumped into the brain, then the brain can no longer be supplied with sufficient energy. The consequences are then movement disorders (dyskinesias) or epileptic seizures, which can occur with the smallest stimuli. Even stimuli such as physical or mental exertion are sufficient to trigger an epileptic seizure. The only way out of this type of disease is fasting. The brain changes its energy supply in such a way that it no longer obtains its energy from sugar (glucose), but from the breakdown products of fats (ketones). This is exactly what happens when you fast long enough. The brain then receives sufficient energy again and is "cured". The epileptic seizures decrease or even normalize.

Today, one falls back again on this therapy form of "fasting" with serious childhood epilepsy forms, by treating the children concerned with a so-called **ketogenic diet**.[182] This ketogenic diet (low-carb diet) is so successful that even in children who have to take **three** to four antiepileptic drugs at the same time in order to be halfway seizure-free, a significant improvement in symptoms can be achieved. Often, a ketogenic diet even achieves freedom from seizures, so that one can speak of a "cure".[183]

Jesus probably used this powerful therapeutic tool unknowingly. Perhaps he observed that (mental) illnesses very often improve through fasting, and therefore brought this therapy into use. In any case, he used it to successfully treat epilepsy and cast out the alleged "evil spirits".

Let us return once again to this "case report" in the Bible. Here there is another interesting passage. It is written that in the case of the child, "the evil spirit has often tried to throw the child into the fire or water and thus kill him". Now, accidents are actually the greatest danger for epileptics because they can fall and injure themselves every time they have a seizure. If they thereby fall into the water and drown or fall into the fire and burn, then this may have been interpreted in biblical times as an "attempt by an evil spirit to destroy the child". What is more interesting here is that the probability of having an epileptic seizure increases in the vicinity of flickering fire or a lake glistening in sunlight. The probability of a seizure increases with repeated light stimuli, as is the case when looking at "flickering flames" or when looking at a "glittering lake". So it is understandable that the boy in the Bible apparently has had seizures several times from such light stimuli, a condition also known as

---

182 Cornejo VE, Cabello JF, Colombo MC, Raimann EB. Síndrome de deficiencia del transportador de glucosa tipo 1 (SDGLUT-1) tratado con dieta cetogénica. Caso clínico [Glucose transponer type 1 deficiency síndrome (GLUT-1 SD) treated with ketogenic diet. Report of one case]. Rev Med Chil. 2007 May;135(5):631–5. Spanish. doi: https://doi.org/10.4067/s0034-98872007000500011. Epub 2007 Jul 9. PMID: 17657332.

183 Winesett SP, Bessone SK, Kossoff EH. The ketogenic diet in pharmacoresistant childhood epilepsy. Expert Rev Neurother. 2015 Jun;15(6):621–8. doi: https://doi.org/10.1586/14737175.2015.1044982. Epub 2015 May 20. PMID: 25994046.

photosensitive epilepsy.[184] It is possible that, when Jesus coaxed the boy into a quiet place, away from triggers for further seizures (like flickering fires and glistening water). He protected the boy from further signs of epilepsy during the rest of that day. That alone would have been enough to convince many people that Jesus had miraculously driven out the evil spirit haunting the boy. If the boy then fasted, as advised, his improvement may have become lasting.

Even today, the same phenomenon is seen in epileptics, especially when they are poorly adjusted. The only difference is that in our time the triggering light stimuli are not blazing flames or a glittering water surface, but **flashes of light on television, in discotheques or in traffic**. How little it is known that flashing light can trigger epileptic seizures can be seen in the development of modern warning lights in road traffic. Every construction site, every new emergency vehicle, every modern construction vehicle is no longer equipped with [steady]warning lights as in the past, but with flashing ones. These greatly increase the risk of people having seizures in road traffic. Such developments greatly increase the risk of accidents, and so should actually be replaced by non-flashing ones. Nothing is more dangerous in road traffic than a road user who has an epileptic seizure. But this should only be mentioned in passing. Technicians, designers, and lawyers could still learn something from this case report from the Bible.

Abstract: **Generalized idiopathic epilepsy** (ICD-10: G40.3) with **grand Mal seizures** (ICD-10: G40.6), possibly on the ground of **glucose transporter type 1 deficiency syndrome** (GLUT1-DS), and evidence of **photosensitive epilepsy**.

Variations in the Translation Often Result in Completely Different Content

- In the German Bible translations, Mk 9,29 is always translated approximately as follows: "29 He answered them: This kind can be cast out only by prayer". The word fasting is not used here, while in the other translations (Italian, Latin) it is translated as "He answered them: This kind can be cast out only through prayer and fasting". Here are the original texts:
  - English: English Standard version (Matthew 17, 14–15): 14 And when they came to the crowd, a man came up to him and, kneeling before him, said, "Lord, have mercy on my son, for he has seizures and he suffers terribly. For often he falls into the fire, and often into the water.
  - English: King James Version (Mark 9:28–29): 28 And when he was come into the house, his disciples asked him privately, Why could not we cast him out? 29 And he said unto them, This kind can come forth by nothing, but by prayer and fasting.

---

[184] Poleon S, Szaflarski JP. Photosensitivity in generalized epilepsies. Epilepsy Behav. 2017 Mar;68:225–233. doi: https://doi.org/10.1016/j.yebeh.2016.10.040. Epub 2017 Feb 16. PMID: 28215998.

- Italian: La Parola è Vita (Mark 9,28–29): 28 Poi Gesù entro in una casa con i discepoli, ed essi gli chiesero in privato: "Perché noi non siamo riusciti a cacciare quel demone?" 29 Gesù rispose: "Questo tipo di demoni non si puo mandare via in altro modo, se non con la preghiera e digiuno".
- Latin, Vulgate (Mark 9–27-29): 27 Et cum introisset in domum, discipuli ejus secreto interrogabant eum: Quare nos non potuimus ejicere eum ? 28 Et dixit illis: Hoc genus in nullo potest exire, nisi in oratione et jejunio. 29 Et inde profecti prætergrediebantur Galilæam: nec volebat quemquam scire.

• Also, the passage at Matthew 17,14–15 is translated differently in the German and English translations. While in the German Bible versions it is translated as "moonstruck", in the English translation it is translated as "seizures" which means (epileptic) seizures.

1.28 Jesus Heals a Man Born Blind (The Healing of the Man Born Blind at the Pool of Siloam)

1.28.1 Original Text (John 9:1–41)

Jesus Heals a Man Born Blind (John 9:1–41): 1 As he passed by, he saw a man blind from birth. 2 And his disciples asked him, "Rabbi, who sinned, this man or his parents, that he was born blind?" 3 Jesus answered, "It was not that this man sinned, or his parents, but that the works of God might be displayed in him. 4 We must work the works of him who sent me while it is day; night is coming, when no one can work. 5 As long as I am in the world, I am the light of the world." 6 Having said these things, he spit on the ground and made mud with the saliva. Then he anointed the man's eyes with the mud 7 and said to him, "Go, wash in the pool of Siloam" (which means Sent). So he went and washed and came back seeing. 8 The neighbours and those who had seen him before as a beggar were saying, "Is this not the man who used to sit and beg?" 9 Some said, "It is he." Others said, "No, but he is like him." He kept saying, "I am the man." 10 So they said to him, "Then how were your eyes opened?" 11 He answered, "The man called Jesus made mud and anointed my eyes and said to me, 'Go to Siloam and wash.' So I went and washed and received my sight." 12 They said to him, "Where is he?" He said, "I do not know." 13 They brought to the Pharisees the man who had formerly been blind. 14 Now, it was a Sabbath day when Jesus made the mud and opened his eyes. 15 So the Pharisees again asked him how he had received his sight. And he said to them, "He put mud on my eyes, and I washed, and I see." 16 Some of the Pharisees said, "This man is not from God, for he does not keep the Sabbath." But others said, "How can a man who is a sinner do such signs?" And there was a division among them. 17 So they said again to the blind man, "What do you say about him, since he has opened your eyes?" He said, "He is a prophet." 18 The Jews did not believe that he had been blind and had received his sight, until they called the parents of the man who had received his sight 19 and asked them, "Is this your son, who you say was born blind? How then does he now see?" 20 His parents answered, "We know that this is our son and that he was born blind. 21 But how he now sees we do not know, nor do we know who opened his eyes. Ask him; he is of age. He will speak for himself." 22 (His parents said these things because they feared the Jews, for the Jews had already agreed that if anyone should confess Jesus to be Christ, he was to be put out of the synagogue.) 23 Therefore, his parents said, "He is of age; ask him." 24 So for the second time they called the man who had been blind and said to him, "Give glory to God. We know that this man is a sinner." 25 He answered, "Whether he is a sinner I do not know. One thing I do know, that though I was blind, now I see." 26 They said to him, "What did he do to you? How did he open your eyes?" 27 He answered them, "I have told you already, and you would not listen. Why do you want to hear it again? Do you also want to become his disciples?" 28 And they reviled him, saying, "You are his disciple, but we are disciples of Moses. 29 We know that God has spoken to Moses, but as for this man, we do not know where he comes from." 30 The man answered, "Why, this is an amazing thing! You do not know where he comes from, and yet he opened my eyes. 31 We know that God does not listen to sinners, but if anyone is a worshipper of God and does his will, God listens to him. 32 Never since the world began has it been heard that anyone opened the eyes of a man born blind. 33 If this man were not from God, he could do nothing." 34 They answered him, "You were born in utter sin, and would you teach us?" And they cast him out. 35 Jesus heard that they had cast him out, and having found him, he said, "Do you believe in the Son of Man?" 36 He answered, "And who is he, sir, that I may believe in him?" 37 Jesus said to him, "You have seen him, and it is he who is speaking to you." 38 He said, "Lord, I believe," and he worshipped him. 39 Jesus said, "For judgment I came into this world, that those who do not see may see, and those who see may become blind." 40 Some of the Pharisees near him heard these things, and said to him, "Are we also blind?" 41 Jesus said to them, "If you were blind, you would have no guilt; but now that you say, 'We see,' your guilt remains."

1.28.2 Description and Interpretation

Jesus was staying in Jerusalem with his disciples. As he walked through the city on the Sabbath, he met a beggar who was blind from birth. Then the disciples asked Jesus, "Rabbi, who sinned so that he was born blind, he himself or his parents?" Jesus answered, "Neither he nor his parents sinned, but it came about so that the works of God might be revealed in him". As a result of original sin, all people come into the world imperfect. Therefore, they are not spared infirmities such as blindness. He spat on the ground, made a paste with the saliva and the earth, and spread it on the eyes of the blind man. Then he said, "Go and wash in the pool of Siloam". When the man did this, he could see again. Neighbours and other people who knew him were astonished at this, but others would not believe it and said, "No, he only looks like him". But the man himself affirmed, "It is I". When they asked him how he had regained his sight, he said: Jesus made a paste and put it on my eyes. Then he told me to wash in the pool of Siloam, after which I could see again. There followed an argument with the Pharisees whether it was permissible to heal on the Sabbath.

This story is only found in the Gospel of John. Unfortunately, hardly any additional complaints or symptoms are described, which would allow a more detailed characterization of the clinical picture. Only the description of how the parents reacted to the questioning by the scribes suggests that they were not very caring, and the blind man might not have had a good relationship with his family. In any case, their answer was quite unkind towards their son. Therefore, we can assume that **he did not have much social support in his family, which of course made him more susceptible to psychosomatic processes.**[185]

The Bible speaks of congenital blindness. The layman may imagine this to mean complete blindness, in which those affected can no longer see anything at all or distinguish light from dark. The fact is, however, that most people "born blind" still have certain visual abilities. So light and dark, outlines or even still pictures can be recognized. Such a form of "blindness" is to be assumed also in the biblical case, because people born completely blind have even today in countries of the Third World only very few chances to reach adulthood.[186]

If outlines or pictures could still be recognized, one would speak rather of a severe weak-sightedness or amblyopia.[187] Mostly, this amblyopia is not based on recognizable organic causes,[188] which means that the structures necessary for sharp vision are not diseased. Causes of such amblyopia: Clouding of the lens (cataract),[189] disturbance of the curvature of the lens or the cornea (astigmatism),[190] severe short-sightedness or long-sightedness (myopia or hyperopia)[191] or a **squinting eye (strabismus)**[192] are possible. Especially in the latter case, the affected person is no longer able to bring the images from both eyes to coincide in his brain. By covering one eye, e.g. with saliva and soil, the affected person can see again with one eye. This kind of therapy is often done today with children by covering their glasses so that the child is forced to train the eye that sees worse and then enables the child to bring the images of both eyes to coincide in the brain again. This also makes the strabismus better.

---

[185] Engel GL. The clinical application of the biopsychosocial model. Am J Psychiatry. 1980 May;137(5):535–44. doi: https://doi.org/10.1176/ajp.137.5.535. PMID: 7369396.

[186] Solebo AL, Teoh L, Rahi J. Epidemiology of blindness in children. Arch Dis Child. 2017 Sep;102(9):853–857. doi: https://doi.org/10.1136/archdischild-2016-310532. Epub 2017 May 2. Erratum in: Arch Dis Child. 2017 Oct;102(10):995. PMID: 28465303.

[187] DeSantis D. Amblyopia. Pediatr Clin North Am. 2014 Jun;61(3):505–18. doi: https://doi.org/10.1016/j.pcl.2014.03.006. Epub 2014 Apr 14. PMID: 24852148.

[188] Maurer D, McKEE SP. Classification and diversity of amblyopia. Vis Neurosci. 2018 Jan;35:E012. doi: https://doi.org/10.1017/S0952523817000190. PMID: 29905124.

[189] Mansouri B, Stacy RC, Kruger J, Cestari DM. Deprivation amblyopia and congenital hereditary cataract. Semin Ophthalmol. 2013 Sep–Nov;28(5–6):321–6. doi: https://doi.org/10.3109/08820538.2013.825289. PMID: 24138041.

[190] Harvey EM. Development and treatment of astigmatism-related amblyopia. Optom Vis Sci. 2009 Jun;86(6):634–9. doi: https://doi.org/10.1097/OPX.0b013e3181a6165f. PMID: 19430327; PMCID: PMC2706277.

[191] Barrett BT, Bradley A, Candy TR. The relationship between anisometropia and amblyopia. Prog Retin Eye Res. 2013 Sep;36:120–58. doi: https://doi.org/10.1016/j.preteyeres.2013.05.001. Epub 2013 Jun 15. PMID: 23773832; PMCID: PMC3773531.

[192] Granet DB, Khayali S. Amblyopia and strabismus. Pediatr Ann. 2011 Feb;40(2):89–94. doi: https://doi.org/10.3928/00904481-20110117-08. PMID: 21323205.

The **eye muscles have a very high energy requirement**.[193] Everyone can see this when people who are very tired start to squint slightly and thus inwardly "give up" bringing their images into alignment. Artists have often used this slight squint—also called **esophoria or latent squint** in medicine to represent the state of "transfiguration" when depicting saints, by depicting the figures or images with a slight squint. This was to express that someone is "enraptured", that is, lives in a "different world". In any case, the **function of the eyes also has something to do with exhaustion or courage and confidence**. So a certain psychosomatic component seems to be probable. With courage and confidence, in the short term, it may be more likely to bring the images of both eyes to coincide and to improve the weak vision to some extent. **Possibly this was already enough to interpret this as a miracle**. In any case, it is striking that Jesus did not shy away from touching the sick man, who with his handicap was probably considered a "leper". He was not afraid of social impurity. This alone can mobilize enormous self-healing powers, whatever the cause may have been.

But one can also interpret this biblical passage as a metaphor. The story of the healing of the blind can also be used as a dualism of the terms "being blind" and "being able to see", in a figurative sense.

But the most important statement in this story is that **Jesus clearly rejects the widespread view that disability, suffering or illness is a "punishment from God" for sins committed**. The disciples asked him whether the blame for the person's poor eyesight lay with himself or with his parents. He answers this question about the cause with a "neither nor". Even today, many people believe that **illness is a "punishment" from God**. "What have I done to be punished like this?" are phrases often heard from sick people. Jesus gives a clear answer to this question, namely "nothing".

Abstract: Possible congenital amblyopia (ICD-10 H53.0).

1.29 A Woman with a Disabling Spirit (The Healing of the Woman with the Spirit of Weakness, Healing of a Woman on the Sabbath)

1.29.1 Original Text (Luke 13:10–17)

> **A Woman with a Disabling Spirit (Luke 13:10–17):** 10 Now he was teaching in one of the synagogues on the Sabbath. 11 And behold, there was a woman who had had a disabling spirit for eighteen years. She was bent over and could not fully straighten herself. 12 When Jesus saw her, he called her over and said to her, "Woman, you are freed from your disability." 13 And he laid his hands on her, and immediately she was made straight, and she glorified God. 14 But the ruler of the synagogue, indignant because Jesus had healed on the Sabbath,

[193] Kisilevsky E, Freund P, Margolin E. Mitochondrial disorders and the eye. Surv Ophthalmol. 2020 May–Jun;65(3):294–311. doi: https://doi.org/10.1016/j.survophthal.2019.11.001. Epub 2019 Nov 27. PMID: 31783046.

said to the people, "There are six days in which work ought to be done. Come on those days and be healed, and not on the Sabbath day." 15 Then the Lord answered him, "You hypocrites! Does not each of you on the Sabbath untie his ox or his donkey from the manger and lead it away to water it? 16 And ought not this woman, a daughter of Abraham whom Satan bound for eighteen years, be loosed from this bond on the Sabbath day?" 17 As he said these things, all his adversaries were put to shame, and all the people rejoiced at all the glorious things that were done by him.

1.29.2 Description and Interpretation

Jesus was teaching in the synagogue on a Sabbath. While doing so, he saw a woman who had been plagued by an (evil) spirit for 18 years and therefore could no longer walk upright. Jesus called the woman to him and told her, "you are delivered from your suffering". Immediately, she straightened up and was apparently well again. The synagogue ruler was outraged that Jesus was performing "treatments" on a Sabbath, which was actually forbidden.

There was a woman who had a "spirit of weakness" for eighteen years and "she was, hunched over and totally unable to straighten up". When one reads such a description, the first thing that comes to mind as a physician is a poor, **listless and severely depressed woman**. Mostly, such people are avoided because the public does not know how to deal with depressed people. Dealing with such people is usually perceived as very unpleasant. Depressives radiate rejection and therefore reap rejection again.[194] This puts them in a vicious cycle of isolation, resulting in even more pronounced depression. Jesus, with his enormous empathy, immediately recognized this and **reached out to her** or laid his hand on her. **In doing so, he successfully broke the cycle of rejection and being rejected**.

Depression leads to tension in the spinal muscles, back pain, low back pain and consequently a curved spine.[195] How many mental processes can have to do with "posture"? It can be experienced through language alone, when we hear phrases such as "keep your posture", "take everything on your shoulders", "be an upright person", "be a bent or broken person", and so on. When we want to encourage someone, we sometimes say "chin up" meaning "don't let yourself down" and again "take a stand". This is exactly what Jesus did by relieving the woman of her suffering, thus encouraging her to walk "uprightly" through life again.

This was obviously not inconvenient for him, because the hypocritical synagogue ruler did not have the real salvation of the visitors of his synagogue in mind, but only the holy scriptures, an attitude that Jesus obviously deeply detested. So he could use

---

[194] Schomerus, Georg. "Ablehnung von Menschen mit schweren psychischen Erkrankungen." Psychotherapeut, vol. 59, no. 3, 1 May 2014, pp. 250–2. doi: https://doi.org/10.1007/s00278-014-1052-6.

[195] Hajihasani A, Rouhani M, Salavati M, Hedayati R, Kahlaee AH. The Influence of Cognitive Behavioral Therapy on Pain, Quality of Life, and Depression in Patients Receiving Physical Therapy for Chronic Low Back Pain: A Systematic Review. PM R. 2019 Feb;11(2):167–176. doi: https://doi.org/10.1016/j.pmrj.2018.09.029. Epub 2019 Feb 11. PMID: 30266349.

the situation well to make clear to the visitors of the synagogue that the **Sabbath is for man and not man for the Sabbath**. The miracle here was not so much the healing of a depression, but that he shook up the people and dared to denounce the practised hypocrisy.

Abstract: Recurrent or persistent depressive disorder (ICD-10 F33.1) with psychogenic vertebral syndrome (ICD-10: F45.0).

1.30 The Death of Lazarus (The Raising of Lazarus)

1.30.1 Original Text (John 11:1–44)

The Death of Lazarus (John 11:1–44): 1 Now a certain man was ill, Lazarus of Bethany, the village of Mary and her sister Martha. 2 It was Mary who anointed the Lord with ointment and wiped his feet with her hair, whose brother Lazarus was ill. 3 So the sisters sent to him, saying, "Lord, he whom you love is ill." 4 But when Jesus heard it, he said, "This illness does not lead to death. It is for the glory of God, so that the Son of God may be glorified through it." 5 Now Jesus loved Martha and her sister and Lazarus. 6 So, when he heard that Lazarus was ill, he stayed two days longer in the place where he was. 7 Then after this he said to the disciples, "Let us go to Judea again." 8 The disciples said to him, "Rabbi, the Jews were just now seeking to stone you, and are you going there again?" 9 Jesus answered, "Are there not twelve hours in the day? If anyone walks in the day, he does not stumble, because he sees the light of this world. 10 But if anyone walks in the night, he stumbles, because the light is not in him." 11 After saying these things, he said to them, "Our friend Lazarus has fallen asleep, but I go to awaken him." 12 The disciples said to him, "Lord, if he has fallen asleep, he will recover." 13 Now Jesus had spoken of his death, but they thought that he meant taking rest in sleep. 14 Then Jesus told them plainly, "Lazarus has died, 15 and for your sake I am glad that I was not there, so that you may believe. But let us go to him." 16 So Thomas, called the Twin, said to his fellow disciples, "Let us also go, that we may die with him."

I Am the Resurrection and the Life: 17 Now when Jesus came, he found that Lazarus had already been in the tomb four days. 18 Bethany was near Jerusalem, about two miles off, 19 and many of the Jews had come to Martha and Mary to console them concerning their brother. 20 So when Martha heard that Jesus was coming, she went and met him, but Mary remained seated in the house. 21 Martha said to Jesus, "Lord, if you had been here, my brother would not have died. 22 But even now I know that whatever you ask from God, God will give you." 23 Jesus said to her, "Your brother will rise again." 24 Martha said to him, "I know that he will rise again in the resurrection on the last day." 25 Jesus said to her, "I am the resurrection and the life. Whoever believes in me, though he die, yet shall he live, 26 and everyone who lives and believes in me shall never die. Do you believe this?" 27 She said to him, "Yes, Lord; I believe that you are the Christ, the Son of God, who is coming into the world."

Jesus Weeps: 28 When she had said this, she went and called her sister Mary, saying in private, "The Teacher is here and is calling for you." 29 And when she heard it, she rose quickly and went to him. 30 Now Jesus had not yet come into the village, but was still in the place where Martha had met him. 31 When the Jews who were with her in the house, consoling her, saw Mary rise quickly and go out, they followed her, supposing that she was going to the tomb to weep there. 32 Now when Mary came to where Jesus was and saw him, she fell at his feet, saying to him, "Lord, if you had been here, my brother would not have died." 33 When Jesus saw her weeping, and the Jews who had come with her also weeping, he was deeply moved[5] in his spirit and greatly troubled. 34 And he said, "Where have you laid him?" They said to him, "Lord, come and see." 35 Jesus wept. 36 So the Jews said, "See how he loved him!" 37 But some of them said, "Could not he who opened the eyes of the blind man also have kept this man from dying?".

Jesus Raises Lazarus: 38 Then Jesus, deeply moved again, came to the tomb. It was a cave, and a stone lay against it. 39 Jesus said, "Take away the stone." Martha, the sister of the dead man, said to him, "Lord, by this time there will be an odor, for he has been dead four days." 40 Jesus said to her, "Did I not tell you that if you believed you would see the glory of God?" 41 So they took away the stone. And Jesus lifted up his eyes and said, "Father, I thank you that you have heard me. 42 I knew that you always hear me, but I said this on account of the people standing around, that they may believe that you sent me." 43 When he had said these things, he cried out with a loud voice, "Lazarus, come out." 44 The man who had died came out, his hands and feet bound with linen strips, and his face wrapped with a cloth. Jesus said to them, "Unbind him, and let him go."

1.30.2 Description and Interpretation

Jesus was visiting his friends, the sisters Martha and Mary and their brother Lazarus, who was apparently sick at the time. After Jesus left the house of the sisters and went on his way in the direction of the Sea of Galilee, the sisters sent for him, because the health of Lazarus had worsened visibly, and they were worried about him. Jesus did not want to return and stayed two more days in the place where the message reached him. Nevertheless, he went back afterwards in order to see after Lazarus and the sisters. On the way back, Mary met him and threw herself at Jesus' feet, lamenting that her brother had died. "If you had stayed with us and not gone away, my brother would surely have survived", were her words. Jesus was greatly affected by the sorrow of the weeping Mary and allowed himself to be led to the tomb of Lazarus. He ordered the tombstone that closed the cave of Lazarus' tomb to be removed. Martha and Mary warned Jesus that Lazarus already smelled of decay, for he had been lying in that tomb for 4 days. Jesus nevertheless insisted that the tomb be opened. He called loudly inside "Lazarus come out". Then the deceased came out wrapped in his linen cloths and bandages. Jesus ordered taking off the bandages and the sweat cloth that covered his face and let Lazarus go.

Let us assume that Lazarus had a serious infection. Then one could assume that it would still take some time before one saw how the illness would develop. Lazarus slept the whole time, which is normal with a serious infection and is also the best way to mobilize the self-healing forces. This may also have been the reason, why Jesus did not return immediately, although his friends Martha and Mary called him for help. If the sick person was hardly responsive and also emitted a foul odour, it is likely that he had a **severe infection with anaerobic or putrid germs**. In most cases, such infections are urinary tract infections[196] or wound infections.[197]

What happened in the case of a severe infection in times when antibiotics were not yet available? In such a case, the body initially ramps up all its performance; Pulse, and respiration increase. Later, the body reduces all performance in order to save energy: Breathing becomes shallow and barely noticeable, pulse becomes weak and barely noticeable and consciousness dulls, and you sleep all the time. The ancient physicians, who still knew the Latin language, spoke of a **"vita minima" or apparent death**.[198] In this case, all life processes are so reduced that they are only detectable by special device-based examination methods such as ECG and EEG.[199] Today, such conditions are rarely seen when a person goes into septic shock. However, such people do not always die! It is easy to imagine that in biblical times, breathing was no longer perceptible, the pulse was no longer palpable, and consciousness was so clouded that the affected person could not be awakened. **In such a condition, the determination of death is really not easy even for medical experts.**[200] If a bad smell is also present, then it is particularly in southern countries high time that such a person should be interred in the grave, also to avoid a spreading of infections. Even today, in southern countries, the deceased must be buried within 24 h. This is a period in which death cannot be determined with absolute certainty. Bad smell is, in any case, not a sure sign of death! Even living people can produce pretty bad smells, especially when they are sick. Anyone who has ever been in a poorly run nursing home will have experienced that it takes your breath away as soon as you enter the building. If any of the many inmates are suffering from an untreated urinary tract or gastrointestinal infection, they can smell quite offensive.

But let us come back to Lazarus once again. The Bible tells us that he was "wrapped with bandages". People used to bandage corpses to keep them from decomposing too quickly. For this purpose, depending on availability, one used in those days, clay, wax, resin, or glue so that the bandages "stuck". The bandages compressed the vessels. If resins were used as glue, then resin acids, tannin acids, and other ingredients could exert their pharmacological effects. Natural resins, for example, are thought to have anti-inflammatory and disinfectant effects (e.g. terpenes).[201] Wax, which was used as an adhesive, is also thought to have a number of pharmacologically active substances

[196] Is malodorous urine associated with urinary tract infection in children? J Paediatr Child Health. 2012 Oct;48(10):945–6. https://doi.org/10.1111/j.1440-1754.2012.02563.x. PMID: 23094623.

[197] Ousey K, Roberts D, Gefen A. Early identification of wound infection: understanding wound odour. J Wound Care. 2017 Oct 2;26(10):577–582. doi: https://doi.org/10.12968/jowc.2017.26.10.577. PMID: 28976829.

[198] Gütgemann A, Käufer C. Der Scheintod [Apparent death]. Dtsch Med Wochenschr. 1970 Mar 27;95(13):702–6. German. doi: https://doi.org/10.1055/s-0028-1108530. PMID: 5437138.

[199] DocCheck Medical Services GmbH. "Scheintod - DocCheck Flexikon." DocCheck Flexikon, 27 Nov. 2021, flexikon.doccheck.com/de/Scheintod.

[200] Schirmer H. Skinndøden. Folketro og realitet [Apparent death. Popular belief and reality]. Tidsskr Nor Laegeforen. 1974 Nov 10;94(31):2135–9. Norwegian. PMID: 4610893.

[201] Simpson BS, Luo X, Wang J, Song Y, Claudie D, Garg S, Smith N, McKinnon R, Semple S. Development and Evaluation of a Topical Anti-Inflammatory Preparation Containing Dodonaea

(e.g. propolis) that exerted an effect by passing through the skin into the body.[202] In any case, the compression of the vessels had a circulatory stabilizing effect.

All this was certainly not known at that time, but it certainly worked. In addition, the "dead person" was moved to the burial place. Presumably it was much cooler there than it was in his own home. That could lead once again to the fact that the circulation situation could improve. Oxygen saturation in the lungs also improves when the ambient air is cooler. All in all, not much more could have been done with the conditions of the time to "treat" a terminally ill person, possibly lying down in septic shock. As I said before: You can die from septic shock, but you don't have to. The "resurrection of a dead person" is more likely to have been a lucky spontaneous healing of a person who had previously been seriously ill.

Abstract: Apparent death (ICD-10 R09.1) in sepsis (ICD-10 A41) caused by anaerobic or putrid germs (ICD-10A 49).

1.31 Jesus Cleanses Ten Lepers (The "Healing" of the Ten Lepers)

1.31.1 Original Text (Luke 17:11–19)

> **Jesus Cleanses Ten Lepers (Luke 17:11–19):** 11 On the way to Jerusalem he was passing along between Samaria and Galilee. 12 And as he entered a village, he was met by ten lepers, who stood at a distance 13 and lifted up their voices, saying, "Jesus, Master, have mercy on us." 14 When he saw them he said to them, "Go and show yourselves to the priests." And as they went, they were cleansed. 15 Then one of them, when he saw that he was healed, turned back, praising God with a loud voice; 16 and he fell on his face at Jesus' feet, giving him thanks. Now he was a Samaritan. 17 Then Jesus answered, "Were not ten cleansed? Where are the nine? 18 Was no one found to return and give praise to God except this foreigner?" 19 And he said to him, "Rise and go your way; your faith has made you well."

1.31.2 Description and Interpretation

Jesus was walking to Jerusalem. When he came to a village, ten leprous men met him. At that time, lepers, who were considered unclean, were commanded to call out "we are unclean" to everyone they met, even from a distance. So the men also called out to Jesus from afar: "Jesus, dear Master, have mercy on us". After Jesus apparently saw that there was no longer any reason for these ten men to be considered

---

polyandra Extract. J Pharm Pharm Sci. 2015;18(4):578–99. doi: https://doi.org/10.18433/j38p57. PMID: 26626250.

[202] Nakao R, Senpuku H, Ohnishi M, Takai H, Ogata Y. Effect of topical administration of propolis in chronic periodontitis. Odontology. 2020 Oct;108(4):704–714. doi: https://doi.org/10.1007/s10266-020-00500-4. Epub 2020 Feb 28. PMID: 32112365.

unclean, he asked them to go to the priests and show them that they were actually no longer unclean. They did so and were found clean by the priests. One of these ten men was so grateful for this that he turned back and threw himself on his knees before Jesus and thanked him for his help. Jesus was pleased, but he asked where the other nine men had gone and if these men had not found it necessary to thank him for his helpful advice.

As stated earlier, leprosy does not mean disease, but a legal status similar to quarantine in modern times. Leprosy could be pronounced by priests according to the rules in the third book of Moses (Leviticus 13) and could also be cancelled (Leviticus14). There the circumstances were exactly described, under which the status of "leprosy" could be imposed and/or lifted again. If people were declared lepers, they lost many rights and were no longer allowed to be near others. Skin lesions were a common reason for declaring someone a "leper". Since lepers were not allowed to go near other people, they often could not even prove that, for example, the skin lesions were no longer present. It was therefore almost impossible to regain the status of "purity" without external help. Jesus helped these men to do this and apparently reaped little thanks for it.

It should be pointed out again: Deliverance from leprosy has nothing to do with healing, but only regaining a normal legal status. The biblical stories that show that lepers were instantly healed of disease are simply false. See also miracle #11.

Abstract: Change the legal status of "being a leper" by Jesus asking the ten men to show themselves to the priests and point out to them that the conditions for the imposition of "leper status" no longer exist.

1.32 Jesus Heals a Blind Beggar (The Healing of Blind Bartimaeus the Blind Man at the Exit of Jericho)

1.32.1 Original Text (Luke 18:35–43; Mark 10:46–52; Matthew 20:29–34)

Jesus Heals a Blind Beggar (Luke 18:35–43): 35 As he drew near to Jericho, a blind man was sitting by the roadside begging. 36 And hearing a crowd going by, he inquired what this meant. 37 They told him, "Jesus of Nazareth is passing by." 38 And he cried out, "Jesus, Son of David, have mercy on me!" 39 And those who were in front rebuked him, telling him to be silent. But he cried out all the more, "Son of David, have mercy on me!" 40 And Jesus stopped and commanded him to be brought to him. And when he came near, he asked him, 41 "What do you want me to do for you?" He said, "Lord, let me recover my sight." 42 And Jesus said to him, "Recover your sight; your faith has made you well." 43 And immediately he recovered his sight and followed him, glorifying God. And all the people, when they saw it, gave praise to God.

Jesus Heals Blind Bartimaeus (Mark 10:46–52): 46 And they came to Jericho. And as he was leaving Jericho with his disciples and a great crowd, Bartimaeus, a blind beggar, the son of Timaeus, was sitting by the roadside. 47 And when he heard that it was Jesus of

Nazareth, he began to cry out and say, "Jesus, Son of David, have mercy on me!" 48 And many rebuked him, telling him to be silent. But he cried out all the more, "Son of David, have mercy on me!" 49 And Jesus stopped and said, "Call him." And they called the blind man, saying to him, "Take heart. Get up; he is calling you." 50 And throwing off his cloak, he sprang up and came to Jesus. 51 And Jesus said to him, "What do you want me to do for you?" And the blind man said to him, "Rabbi, let me recover my sight." 52 And Jesus said to him, "Go your way; your faith has made you well." And immediately he recovered his sight and followed him on the way.

Jesus Heals Two Blind Men (Matthew 20:29–34): 29 And as they went out of Jericho, a great crowd followed him. 30 And behold, there were two blind men sitting by the roadside, and when they heard that Jesus was passing by, they cried out, "Lord,[5] have mercy on us, Son of David!" 31 The crowd rebuked them, telling them to be silent, but they cried out all the more, "Lord, have mercy on us, Son of David!" 32 And stopping, Jesus called them and said, "What do you want me to do for you?" 33 They said to him, "Lord, let our eyes be opened." 34 And Jesus in pity touched their eyes, and immediately they recovered their sight and followed him.

1.32.2 Description and Interpretation

When Jesus came to Jericho, a blind man was sitting by the roadside begging. The blind man noticed that many people were passing by. He asked what was going on and was told that Jesus of Nazareth was passing by. The blind man called out to Jesus, "Son of David, have mercy on me". The people who went ahead ordered the blind man to be silent, but he cried out even more loudly to Jesus, asking him to help him. Then the blind man jumped up and ran toward Jesus. Jesus asked him what he wanted from him. The blind man answered that he wanted to be able to see again, to which Jesus replied, "be able to see". At the same moment, he could see again.

There are not-so-rare people who cannot see, although their visual apparatus is perfectly fine. That is, the eyes, optic nerves and visual cortex in the brain are perfectly fine, but an unknown process in the brain prevents the affected person from seeing anything. This form of blindness is classified as a **dissociative disorder**[203] and was formerly also called **hysterical blindness** or **conversion neurotic blindness**. One ophthalmologist described the disorder as follows: "When you have to see something you can't stand, there is a way out, which is **psychogenic blindness**".[204] The essential feature of psychogenic blindness is that it is reversible after psychotherapeutic treatment.[205]

Regardless of the fact that psychogenic blindness exists, in the present case the **"blind man" could not really have been completely blind**, otherwise he would

---

[203] Spiegel D, Lewis-Fernández R, Lanius R, Vermetten E, Simeon D, Friedman M. Dissociative disorders in DSM-5. Annu Rev Clin Psychol. 2013;9:299–326. doi: https://doi.org/10.1146/annurev-clinpsy-050212-185531. Epub 2013 Feb 1. PMID: 23394228.

[204] Pohlmann-Eden, B., et al. "Psychogene Blindheit." Aktuelle Neurologie, vol. 20, no. 02, Apr. 1993, pp. 58–61. doi: https://doi.org/10.1055/s-2007-1018001.

[205] Strasburger H, Waldvogel B. Sight and blindness in the same person: Gating in the visual system. Psych J. 2015 Dec;4(4):178–85. doi: https://doi.org/10.1002/pchj.109. Epub 2015 Oct 15. PMID: 26468893.

not have been able to jump up and run to Jesus. Furthermore, it is remarkable in the described story that the "blind beggar" must have been from a "good family". Nobody would have known his name otherwise, let alone the name of his father, if he had been a "real beggar". Beggars were (and unfortunately still are) considered "non-persons" and are rarely called by name, much less by their father's name. Moreover, he seemed to have been aloof and somewhat insolent, shouting so loudly that other people were embarrassed and wanted to keep him away from Jesus. All of these features point to a badly neglected person and also fit a dissociative disorder.[206]

In 2015, a case report of psychogenic blindness in a young woman was described.[207] In this case, the blindness was even preceded by psychogenic aphonia ("it made her lose her voice") and psychogenic paralysis ("when someone is as if paralysed"). Arriving at the eye clinic, she was blind, but objectively no visual disturbance could be detected. The problems of the psychologically "unremarkable" 21-year-old student arose after her father became seriously ill, which was associated with the fear that she would not be able to finish her studies. After psychotherapeutic treatment, she was "miraculously" cured. One can see from this case report beautifully what complex complaints dissociative disorders can entail and that psychogenic blindness is still topical, as are psychogenic paralysis and psychogenic muteness.

Abstract: Dissociative Sensory Disorders (ICD-1: F44.6). The usual translation of this Bible passage is very questionable. It does not give sufficient information to make an interpretation of a miracle healing possible.

[206] Choi KR, Seng JS, Briggs EC, Munro-Kramer ML, Graham-Bermann SA, Lee RC, Ford JD. The Dissociative Subtype of Posttraumatic Stress Disorder (PTSD) Among Adolescents: Co-Occurring PTSD, Depersonalization/Derealization, and Other Dissociation Symptoms. J Am Acad Child Adolesc Psychiatry. 2017 Dec;56(12):1062–1072. doi: https://doi.org/10.1016/j.jaac.2017.09.425. Epub 2017 Oct 4. PMID: 29173740; PMCID: PMC5726572.

[207] S. Mulugeta, K. Tesfay, R. Frank, and C. Gruber-Frank. Acute Loss of Vision in a Young Woman: A Case Report on Psychogenic Blindness, Ethiop J Health Sci. 2015 Jan; 25(1): 99–104. PMCID: PMC4337078; PMID: 25733790.

Chapter 2
Diseases Commonly Found in the Bible

Since it is not easy for the nonmedical person to understand how sudden healings can occur, I would like to describe here some clinical pictures that occur several times in the Bible. Especially in the case of psychiatric illnesses, spontaneous healings are often particularly impressive because they can often take place immediately and are thus clearly visible to those around them. The best way to imagine this is that when someone gives good news to a sad person, the sadness can evaporate quickly. A "sudden spontaneous healing" has occurred, so to speak. Although there are also spontaneous healings in internal diseases (e.g. tumours), the success does not usually occur suddenly. In the case of psychiatric diseases, a doctor who radiates calmness, sovereignty, and competence can achieve such a strong placebo effect by his presence or appearance alone that (almost) all complaints suddenly disappear. Yes, just the announcement that a doctor is coming, or that competent help is in prospect can lead to spontaneous healing (e.g. toothache that fades away as soon as you get the dentist's appointment). In a way, the doctor becomes a "drug", as Balint has described it several times. The helping person gets a placebo function, so to speak. Outsiders perceive "miraculous" healings in this way, although they are not miracles.

2.1 Diseases That May Suddenly Stop

It is particularly impressive to see someone suddenly healed, e.g. when someone goes bent over to a physiotherapist and the latter frees the pain-ridden person with a jerk, whereas many doctors had failed to improve the condition. Even today, one reads again and again about miracle healings in the Philippines, diseases where conventional medicine has failed, brought about by physicians, therapists or practical men with "golden hands" and other miraculous healers, to whom one should go for healing.

M. Ledochowski, *The Miracles of the Bible Viewed Differently*,
https://doi.org/10.1007/978-3-031-51639-9_2

The failure of conventional medicine in such cases is usually related to the fact that medicine is too specialized. The specialist does his work, and may be good in his field, but the more he specializes, the less knowledge he has about other diseases. Especially when it comes to psychiatric diseases, the knowledge of doctors from other specialities is often poor. Thus, it may well happen that even today, patients run from doctor to doctor for a long time and never find the right one. Finally, they end up with an alternative practitioner. Since the latter has a much lower level of medical training, he can see the person more "holistically" and therefore recognizes a psychological ailment sooner than the highly specialized professor. He responds to this person, takes him seriously, listens to his concerns and is not in a hurry. Simply through such empathetic responsiveness, which the person in question may never have experienced before, a spontaneous, even sudden cure can occur. Here are some examples of such diseases, which are also described in the Bible.

2.1.1 Anxiety Disorders, Panic Attacks and Hyperventilation Syndrome

For the layman, it is most difficult to understand or believe that Jesus or any human being can heal someone within seconds or minutes. This is understandable. Personally, I would not have believed in it if I had not experienced such healing successes within a few minutes.

The most impressive healing successes can be experienced with panic attacks that are accompanied by hyperventilation syndrome. The affected person offers a rather dramatic performance to onlookers. People present often believe that the affected person will die right now if competent help does not come immediately. For people present who have to witness something like this, the situation is almost always an extraordinary burden, especially since no one knows how to react. If such a hyperventilation syndrome lasts for a longer period of time, the fear is frequently transferred to the observers. This creates a social interaction in which not only the panic attack in the first affected person is worsened, but it can even happen that others nearby also develop panic attacks. Personally, I have experienced how a mother developed a panic attack with hyperventilation tetany in reaction to her daughter's panic attack. By the time the ambulance arrived at the emergency room, the condition was so bad that not only the daughter but also her mother had to be treated.

There are an incredible number of people who suffer from anxiety. It is assumed that today, about every third person experiences at least one episode of an anxiety disorder or even a panic attack once in their life.[1] Even today, such episodes are often not recognized. One notices a peculiar, often restless behaviour in those affected. If

[1] Bandelow B, Michaelis S. Epidemiology of anxiety disorders in the 21st century. Dialogues Clin Neurosci. 2015 Sep;17(3):327–35. doi: https://doi.org/10.31887/DCNS.2015.17.3/bbandelow. PMID: 26487813; PMCID: PMC4610617.

the physical reactions are strong, the family typically speaks of a "nervous breakdown" or "hysterical attack" or makes other derogatory statements. In addition to sweating, rapid heartbeat, dizziness, nausea and numerous other vegetative symptoms, a panic attack frequently results in a so-called hyperventilation syndrome[2] with acute shortness of breath (see box). Even today, the symptom "hyperventilation" frequently remains unrecognized.

Hyperventilation means "breathing too much". The purpose behind this increase in breathing is to supply the body with more oxygen and thus prepare it for an emergency. So when someone completes a 100 m run, they consume more oxygen than they can breathe in during that time. This creates what is known as an "oxygen debt", which is made up for by the person breathing faster. This type of hyperventilation, in which one breathes faster, is usually readily apparent. We then speak of someone who "gets out of breath" after an effort or when excited. Less well known is another form of hyperventilation, which occurs mainly as a preparation for emergencies. In this case, the affected person does not breathe noticeably faster, but deeper. This change in breathing is hardly noticed by people nearby. As a result, more energy is made available to the body and reactions such as flight or fight are more possible. This second type of hyperventilation occurs frequently, especially during fear and panic reactions. Subjectively, this form of hyperventilation is experienced as shortness of breath. Objectively, one hardly sees any of it, except that the affected person feels very bad.

Hyperventilation syndrome: In the context of hyperventilation, there are often very unpleasant side effects, which in their entirety are referred to as hyperventilation syndrome.

Increased breathing increases the intake of oxygen, but at the same time the body also loses a lot of carbon dioxide quickly, and this has dramatic consequences. If you breathe out too much CO_2, the pH value in the blood shifts. The blood becomes more alkaline, with the result that divalent ions such as calcium or magnesium are bound to the protein molecules present in the blood. As a result, these ions are no longer available to the nerves in sufficient quantities. The nerves start to "go crazy". The first symptoms appear, especially where there are a lot of nerve endings. There are tingling sensations in the hands, the feet and sometimes also in the face. This is perceived by the affected person as very unpleasant and very often frightening. As a result, sufferers become even more anxious. Anxiety can not only trigger hyperventilation, but also intensify it. As it progresses, the function of the nerves is disturbed even more. A vicious circle develops: anxiety leads to hyperventilation, and hyperventilation leads to anxiety. Thus, after some time, not only dysfunction of the sensory

[2] Du Pasquier D, Fellrath JM, Sauty A. Syndrome d'hyperventilation et respiration dysfonctionnelle: mise à jour [Hyperventilation syndrome and dysfunctional breathing : update]. Rev Med Suisse. 2020 Jun 17;16(698):1243–1249. French. PMID: 32558453.

nerves with **paresthesia**, but also muscle cramps and paralysis occur because the function of the motor nerves is also disturbed. Since mainly hands and feet are affected, one also speaks of **carpopedal spasms.** If not only hands and feet cramp, but more extensive paralysis symptoms occur, one speaks of hyperventilation tetany.

After more and more nerve plexuses no longer fulfil their function due to the functional calcium and magnesium deficiency, more complex disorders can arise eventually. The mimic musculature no longer functions. The affected person gets a **grimace-like appearance**. The muscles that supply the vocal cords no longer do their job, so the familiar **voice can change to a frightening degree**. Such voice changes may be interpreted by outsiders who have to witness something like this as the "voice of the devil or demons". Finally, perceptual disturbances also occur. Sufferers may experience **hallucinations** and see, hear, smell or feel things that are not there.

In the context of hyperventilation syndrome, people often start screaming and thus put others in fear and terror. In such situations, bystanders usually react with pronounced helplessness. This in turn increases the fear of the affected person even more because they realize that no one can help them. Sometimes, entire groups of people can thus go into a panic reaction and behave quite strangely. That can take on quite dramatic proportions and lead to **mass panic** or **mass psychosis**.

Recovery from hyperventilation syndrome occurs at the latest when the affected person becomes unconscious. The anxiety then subsides, breathing levels off again, the pH value in the blood returns to normal and the nerves resume their normal function. Such "healing processes" can be accelerated if someone comes and radiates calmness or sovereignty. Someone who will lay on hands or gives orders and thus distracts the patient from the exciting situation. In today's clinical routine, the appearance of the doctor is often enough for the whole affair to calm down again. From this viewpoint, a doctor can work "miracles" just by his appearance. The mere prospect of healing can bring about actual healing. The well-known physician Balint also spoke of the "doctor" drug in such cases.

The often described change of voices during so-called possession, as they are often shown in Hollywood movies, can be explained by disturbances of the neuromuscular transmission of the vocal cord muscles. When the muscles of the larynx no longer function properly, there is either a slackening or a particular tension of the larynx. As a result, the voice suddenly becomes unnaturally low or unusually high. In any case, bystanders are startled when the affected person no longer speaks with a familiar voice. This may also be a reason why patients with hyperventilation tetany have also been interpreted as "possessed by a demon".

Bible passages in which hyperventilation may have played a role

- Jesus Heals a Paralytic (Luke 5:17–26); no. 12.
- A Man with a Withered Hand (Luke 6:6–10): No. 13.
- Jesus Heals a Woman and Jairus's Daughter (Luke 8:41–56): No. 20.
- Jesus Walks on the Water (Mark 6:45–52; Matthew 14:22–33; John 6:16–21); no. 23.

For a physician, the Bible reads like a book of medical case reports from ancient times. Above all, one finds descriptions of psychiatric diseases. Many of these diseases that we know today already existed in biblical times. The clinical picture has hardly changed since then, but the view of various diseases has become quite different because today we understand many things that were not understood even a few decades ago. For this reason, we will take a closer look at some of the diseases that occur frequently in the Bible and whose healing was described as a miracle.

For the nonmedical person, it is often not easy to understand how sudden healings can occur. Especially in the case of psychiatric illnesses, spontaneous healings are particularly impressive because they can take place immediately and are thus easily visible to everyone. One can perhaps imagine the healing of a psychiatric illness with the following example: Think of a person with reactive depression, for example, a father who has lost his son and cannot get over his death. He has been feeling depressed for years, lives a withdrawn life, can no longer feel joy or laugh. Nowadays, such a condition would be called a prolonged grief reaction or reactive depression. When this sad person is suddenly given the unexpected news that his son is alive and unharmed at the front door, the sadness may vanish in one fell swoop. A "sudden miraculous spontaneous healing" has occurred, so to speak.

The story of the lost (and possibly dead) son (Luke 15:24) could be such an example. One might argue that this was not a disease, but only worries that had tormented this father. But such stressful situations are the precursors of diseases. The transition from discomfort to illness is a fluid one, and even in our time it is difficult to judge in which stage of an illness someone is. For example, stress can only minimally cloud vision, in that someone's vision becomes progressively worse over the course of a day due to fatigue. In the maximum variant, however, stress can even lead to blindness as part of a dissociative reaction, although from an ophthalmologic point of view no "fault" can be determined.

However, there are also spontaneous healings in non-psychiatric diseases, e.g. in case of a malignant tumour. In these cases, however, spontaneous healing does not start suddenly. In the case of mental illnesses, a doctor who radiates calmness, sovereignty, and competence can achieve such a strong placebo effect by his presence alone that the complaints suddenly disappear. Yes, the mere announcement that a doctor is coming, or that competent help is in prospect, can lead to spontaneous healing.[3]

---

[3] Muench J. Balint work and the creation of medical knowledge. Int J Psychiatry Med. 2018 Jan–Mar;53(1–2):15–23. doi: https://doi.org/10.1177/0091217417745288. Epub 2017 Dec 13. PMID: 29235408.

2.1.2 Dissociative Disorders (Conversion Neuroses)

When someone has experienced something terrible, it usually does not remain without consequences. Sleep disturbances, constantly recurring thoughts of the traumatic situation (flash backs), depression, anxiety disorders and many other complaints may occur. If these complaints last longer than eight weeks, it is called post-traumatic stress disorder (PTSD). Sometimes, however, the injuries are so great (or the resources of the affected person, which would be necessary to process such injuries, are so meagre) that very pronounced processing disorders occur, which are then called *dissociative disorders.* In this case, memories or entire personality parts are "split off". In this way, unbearable experiences can be blocked out, so to speak. Even today, dissociative disorders are often not recognized as such. A dissociative disorder is therefore usually but not always preceded by a mental or physical trauma.

Traumas that can lead to the triggering of dissociative disorders are:

- Rape, sexual violence, sexual abuse,
- torture, murder, manslaughter,
- Combat, war, flight, migration,
- Loss of a loved one, abandonment,
- neglect, abuse.

Reactions in dissociative disorder can vary widely. Typically, there are pseudoneurological manifestations. The affected person may erase any memory of the incident from his or her mind (dissociative amnesia). Perhaps he or she runs somewhere and is not even aware of this escape (dissociative fugue). Or there may be paralysis (dissociative stupor), seizures (dissociative, convulsive seizures). But it can also be that someone goes blind (psychogenic blindness) or deaf (psychogenic deafness) or falls silent (mutism, psychogenic muteness). Feelings of complete absence or possession can also occur after severe traumatic experiences (dissociative trance, "feeling possessed by a demon or power"), etc.

Mild forms of such symptoms have been experienced by many people, e.g., when in a surprising situation "someone has lost the power of speech". Children stop talking to strangers after such situations (selective mutism) or become mute altogether (mutism). Evidence for milder dissociative sensitivity disorders can be found in the form of idioms in common usage. Equivalents for "dissociative paralysis" can also be found in language, when someone "freezes with fright" or is "as if paralysed" in a difficult situation.

The transition from minimal reaction disorders caused by minimal trauma to the most severe reaction disorders is fluid. In the most severe case, the person "separates" his consciousness, so to speak. It is not I, but someone else who has experienced this. Such states of a "split" consciousness are called *dissociation* in psychiatry. When one's own person is perceived as alien, it is also called *depersonalization.* If the environment is perceived as alien, distorted or dull, this is called *derealization.* The experience of the self or the environment suddenly feels alien.

The intensity of the psychological reactions depends on the intensity of the trauma on the one hand, and on one's own available resources on the other. If one has help, social support, education, wealth, etc., it is easier to process trauma.

Types of dissociative disorders (formerly sometimes called conversion neuroses, ICD-10: F44)

- Dissociative amnesia (F44.0: psychogenic memory loss; after combat, injury, etc.).
- Dissociative fugue (F44.1: ex. Psychogenic running away, often coupled with memory loss).
- Dissociative stupor (F44.2: Absence of voluntary movements; does not respond to external stimuli).
- Trance and possession states (F44.3: loss of personal identity (trance), belief of being ruled by a "power" (possession).
- Movement disorders (F44.4: psychogenic paralysis, vocal cord paralysis(!), most common form of dissociative disorder).
  - Aphonia, dysphonia, dysarthria (loss of voluntary motor function, speech).
  - Dyskinesia, ataxia, incoordination, or inability to stand without assistance.
- Dissociative seizures (F44.5: psychogenic non-epileptic seizures, PNEA).
- Dissociative sensory disorders (F44.6: psychogenic failures of sensory organs even though they are "organically intact")
  - Blindness.
  - Deafness, muteness.
  - Olfactory disorders, etc.
- Dissociative identity disorder (F44.81: feeling that more than one person is living in one).

When rescue or help is in sight, such morbid conditions can disappear rather quickly, if not abruptly. One can well imagine that in ancient times poverty, mistreatment, use of violence by the Roman occupying power, social pressure due to strict religious rules, etc. not only led to social conflicts but also massively traumatized many a person. Escape into a dissociative disorder was sometimes the only way to save oneself from the terrible reality. Dissociative disorders were first described in antiquity by Hippocrates, so they were already known during Christ's lifetime (see box).

Excursus: The term hysteria comes from the Greek. Hippocrates observed dissociative symptoms, especially in women and particularly the globus sensation, which often occurs at the beginning of dissociative events or shortly before a panic attack. He believed that in these women the uterus (Hystera) wanders around in the body, finally getting stuck in the throat and "clogging" the neck there. Thus, the term "hysteria" was born, referring to the "uterus stuck in the throat". You can frequently experience this observation yourself. When children are sad and begin to cry, they typically describe having a "lump feeling" in their throat. In the language, we find the expression "it makes your throat tight".

In the Middle Ages, this symptom was attributed to possession by the devil or malevolent demons. In modern times, J. M. Charcot called hysteria a "somatic nervous disorder". S. Freud spoke of "conversion hysteria" and thus pioneered the term: "conversion neurosis", which was attributed to unresolved conflicts. P. Janet used for the first time the term "splitting off" of certain contents of experience from consciousness, and thus created the term "dissociation".

Dissociative disorders are exclusion diagnoses. This means that before a dissociative disorder can be diagnosed, all organic diseases must first be ruled out. In today's world, this means a great deal of examination, but it ensures that organic functions such as muscles, nerves, sensory organs (vision or hearing) and the brain are completely intact. The perfect functioning of the physical organs also explains why such diseases can be cured instantly. Actually, everything works and is blocked only by a psychological reaction. If the psychic blockage is removed, an instantaneous "healing" can occur. Triggers for such "miracle healings" are circumstances like prospect of redemption by a "saviour" or "healer", affection understanding or simply attention, etc. A good part of psychotherapy today is based on these "miraculous" effects. Even if functions have been blocked for years, it can still lead to spontaneous and sudden healing. Jesus showed in many situations that he combined all the mentioned characteristics. Seen in this way, he had all the prerequisites for an ideal miracle healer.

Retrospectively, in many miraculous healings described in the Bible, one can guess what diseases they might have been. If one knows that such diseases exist and therefore could be possible even 2000 years ago, they are always more probable than real miracles. The disease group of dissociative disorders is predestined for miracle cures, especially since they are by definition psychologically caused and can be cured by psychotherapeutic measures. Any help can work wonders here. Just the appearance of a doctor or the prospect of getting help leads to healing in a miraculous way here in many cases. The more often Jesus was successful, the more effective his future healings will have been.

Miraculous healings in which dissociative disorders may have played a role

- No. 17: The healing of two blind men (Mt 9:27–31).
- No. 18: Healing of a mute man (Lk 11:14–16; Mt 9:32–34).
- No. 25: Healing of the deaf and mute in Decapolis (Mark 7:31–37, Matthew 15:29–31).
- No. 26: The healing of the blind man of Bethsaida (Mark 8:22–26).
- No. 32: The healing of blind Bartimaeus, healing of the blind man at the outskirts of Jericho (Luke 18:35–43; Mark 10:46–52; Matthew 20:29–34).

2.1.2.1 Psychogenic Movement Disorders (Paralyses)

Psychogenic movement disorders are manifested by gait disturbances such as limping, stumbling, restricted movement, hip pain or even complete paralysis.[4] They are generally classified as dissociative disorders (F44.2 or F44.4) but may also occur transiently in the context of a panic attack with hyperventilation tetany. Other names for psychogenic paralysis are "functional movement disorder", "dissociative movement disorder", "hysterical paralysis", "psychosomatic movement disorder", "conversion neurotic paralysis", or "chronic neurosis".[5] Today, 1–2% of all children are affected. In adults, psychogenic movement disorders occur less frequently, especially since in Western countries appropriate therapy is almost always started in childhood so that a psychogenic movement disorder hardly ever remains undetected until adulthood. In ancient times, however, it can be assumed that this type of movement disorder occurred with the same frequency as in children. As with all dissociative diseases, a prerequisite for the diagnosis of a psychogenic movement disorder is that there is no organic disease causally related to it. While today organic disorders can be excluded by clinical neurological as well as technical device-based examinations, this was not possible in biblical times. Only the indications in the Bible that the therapeutic successes were sudden, however, make the diagnosis of a psychogenic movement disorder probable.

Examples of possible psychogenic movement disorders are

- No. 6: Healing of the sick man at the pool of Bethesda (Jn 5:1–9).
- No. 12: healing of a paralytic after forgiveness of sins (Lk 5:17–26, Mk 2:1–12; Mt 9:1–8).
- No. 14: Remote healing of the servant of a Roman officer in Capernaum (Lk 7:1–10; Mt 8:5–13).
- No. 29: Healing of a woman on the Sabbath (Lk 13:10–17).

2.1.2.2 Psychogenic Hearing Disorders (Deafness)

If someone can no longer or no longer wants to hear something ("I can't hear that anymore", "I don't want to hear about that anymore"), it can happen that the brain fails to process what is heard.[6] Those affected then state that they can only hear poorly or no longer hear anything at all. Today, it is possible to determine very

---

[4] Deutscher Ärzteverlag GmbH, Redaktion. "Psychogene Lähmung im Kindes- und Jugendalter: Gute Prognose bei multimodaler Therapie." Deutsches Ärzteblatt, 10 Jan. 2003, www.aerzteblatt.de/archiv/35145/Psychogene-Laehmung-im-Kindes-und-Jugendalter-Gute-Prognose-bei-multimodaler-Therapie.

[5] Jith A, Narayanan D. Dissociative Motor Disorder. Indian J Psychol Med. 2017 Jan-Feb;39(1):99–101. doi: https://doi.org/10.4103/0253-7176.198952. PMID: 28250569; PMCID: PMC5330002.

[6] Diab KM, Sapozhnikov YM, Naumova IV, Sokolova VN, Kapelyush NV, Balakireva OA. Psikhogennoe narushenie slukha u deteĭ i podrostkov [The psychogenic hearing disorders in the children and adolescents]. Vestn Otorinolaringol. 2017;82(5):77–79. Russian. doi: https://doi.org/10.17116/otorino201782577-79. PMID: 29072671.

well with technical devices whether a sound is heard in an examined person and reaches the brain or not. If the hearing and the auditory nerves are intact, but nothing is heard, one must assume a dissociative (conversion neurotic) disorder. In such cases, purely psychological measures can bring about (abrupt) improvement. Other names for this disorder are "functional hearing loss", "non-organic hearing loss", "dissociative sensory disorder with hearing loss", "pseudohypacusis" or "hysterical deafness". Psychogenic hearing disorders occur frequently in combination with other psychiatric disorders such as autism, impulse control disorders, ADHD, depression, anxiety disorder and especially social phobia.[7]

Example of psychogenic hearing disorders

- No. 25: Healing of the deaf and mute in Decapolis (Mk 7:31–37; Mt 15:29–31).

2.1.2.3 Psychogenic Speechlessness (Muteness) and Hearing Disorders (Deafness)

Voice and mood have a lot to do with each other. When you are angry or when you have a mishap, you are "speechless". In the same way, psychological trauma or psychiatric illnesses can cause someone to become speechless. The type of speechlessness can be different. Very shy small children can often be seen hiding behind their parents and not uttering a word to strangers. When this condition becomes more severe, it is called "selective mutism". This means that the children can no longer talk to certain people. Some people are so inhibited that they stop speaking at all so that the mutism is no longer selective but turns into "psychogenic aphonia", i.e. complete speechlessness.

Milder forms are simple voice changes such as hoarseness, which is then called "dissociative dysphonia". What all forms have in common is that the speech organs are actually intact, but speech is not possible. The speech disorder may last only for a short period of time, e.g., short-term silencing due to a shock ("speech impediment"), or it may persist for a longer period of time. The latter form of speech disorder usually develops between the eighth to tenth year of life. The development of such speech disorders is either a result of a developmental disorder or post-traumatic stress disorder (PTSD). Associated symptoms often include compulsive throat clearing and/or sonorous coughing.

Examples of psychogenic speechlessness and hearing disorders are

- No. 2: The announcement of the birth of John the Baptist (Lk 1:5–25).
- No. 18: Healing of a mute man (Lk 11:14–16; Mt 9:32–34).
- No. 25: Healing of the deaf and mute in Decapolis (Mk 7:31–37; Mt 15:29–31).

---

[7] Bailly D, Dechoulydelenclave MB, Lauwerier L. Déficience auditive et troubles psychopathologiques chez l'enfant et l'adolescent [Hearing impairment and psychopathological disorders in children and adolescents. Review of the recent literature]. Encephale. 2003 Jul–Aug;29(4 Pt 1):329–37. French. PMID: 14615703.

2.1.2.4 Psychogenic Visual Disorders (Blindness)

There are people who cannot see anything because their psyche or some other as yet unknown process in the brain prevents them from perceiving what they see. The visual apparatus, consisting of the eyes, the optic nerve and the areas of the brain that process the visual impulses, are physiologically completely intact. This disease is not limited to exotic individual cases, but occurs more frequently than is assumed. How it comes about is still not known. In any case, the affected persons are not malingerers, but actually see nothing. It can range from simple visual deterioration (visual loss) to complete loss of vision. Sometimes there is only a concentric visual field narrowing in both eyes ("tunnel vision"). Always, the reduction of visual ability or the complete loss of visual ability occurs without any organic basis. This type of visual disorder is classified as a dissociative disorder. Other terms are "psychogenic blindness", "dissociative sensitivity disorder", "functional visual disorder", "psychogenic visual loss", "hysterical blindness" or "conversion neurotic blindness". The multitude of terms alone shows that over time this type of visual disorder has been observed repeatedly, but medical professionals have had difficulty assigning it to a specific disease group. Whereas psychogenic blindness used to be assigned to the neuroses (conversion neurosis), today, as mentioned, it is assigned to the dissociative disorders. Almost always, a severe psychological trauma precedes the condition in affected persons.

The neural basis of psychogenic blindness may be a "top-down modulation" of the activity of the primary visual pathway at the level of the thalamus or primary visual cortex. Using visual evoked potentials (so-called VEP examinations), psychogenic blindness cannot be distinguished from organic causes of visual pathway disruption. It seems that psychogenic blindness blocks the inflow of visual information at an early stage. The affected persons are, so to speak, "blind and seeing in one person". How much the psyche is connected with the sense of sight can be seen in expressions such as "someone sees black" or "someone sees red", "someone was blind with rage" etc.

Most often, such psychogenic visual disorders occur in girls between the ages of 10 and 14. Ophthalmologists describe such visual disorders with the words: "The eye works, but the brain does not allow the images". Psychologists assume that unresolved conflicts or traumas, for example war experiences, underlie the blindness. These cause patients to unconsciously block out visual information because they "don't want to see the bad experiences anymore": A study published in the EPMA journal reports that chronic psychological distress may be responsible for vision loss.[8] The problem with this is primarily that not only can stress lead to impaired vision, but conversely, the reduced vision itself can further worsen vision. Thus, a vicious cycle is created: stress can lead to impaired vision, and impaired vision causes stress, so individuals can remain "trapped" in this cycle. Until there is some prospect of "relief" or "cure". There are case reports of how stress initiates vision loss and how

[8] Sabel, B.A., Wang, J., Cárdenas-Morales, L. et al. EPMA Journal (2018) 9:133. https://doi.org/10.1007/s13167-018-0136-8.

reducing stress restores vision. Both the eye and the brain are involved in vision difficulties. For example, increased intraocular pressure, endothelial dysfunction of the blood vessels in the eye (Flammer's syndrome), and inflammatory eye disease can be effects of distress, which in turn can cause further damage.[9]

Stress reduction and imparting calmness and composure was apparently one of Jesus' strengths. Thus, the prerequisite was given to perform an "ophthalmological miracle healing". It is also conceivable, that such psychological relief could improve not only dissociative disorders, but also other conditions affecting visual performance, such as excessive eye pressure associated with glaucoma or optic nerve damage. Visual acuity may also suffer temporarily due to stress: As a result of strong psychological tension, the ciliary muscles to which the lenses are attached tense up so that the eye remains adjusted to near vision. This is called "pseudo-near-sightedness", which is often accompanied by headaches. In addition, there are tangible eye diseases in whose development and course the psyche obviously plays a role. The background is usually complicated, as Emmerich explains: "Unresolved conflicts can cause changes in the autonomic nervous system and hormones and thus promote the development of a disease or prolong its duration".

A typical example is the mysterious eye disease "**Central Serous Chorioretinopathy (CSCR)**",[10] in which fluid accumulates under the central retina. The disease strikingly often affects men between 30 and 50 years of age who are under heavy professional strain, which is why it is also called "manager's disease of the eye". How CSCR develops is unclear. One suspects a connection with the personality of the patients: These frequently show "type A behaviour", that is, they display an increased willingness to perform in competitive situations. This stimulates the autonomic nervous system more strongly, which leads to an increased release of the stress hormone cortisol. This effect could be an important trigger for the disease.

Another disease for which the influence of the psyche has long been speculated is glaucoma, which causes the optic nerve to die. Indeed, psychological strain and stress can alter intraocular pressure, which is considered a risk factor for glaucoma. Conversely, studies have shown that autogenic training and endurance sports have a beneficial effect on intraocular pressure.[11,12]

---

[9] Universitätsklinikum Magdeburg; Sabel, B.A., Wang, J., Cárdenas-Morales, L. et al. EPMA Journal (2018) 9:133. https://doi.org/10.1007/s13167-018-0136-8.

[10] Sesar AP, Sesar A, Bucan K, Sesar I, Cvitkovic K, Cavar I. Personality Traits, Stress, and Emotional Intelligence Associated with Central Serous Chorioretinopathy. Med Sci Monit. 2021 Jan 10;27:e928677. doi: https://doi.org/10.12659/MSM.928677. PMID: 33423036; PMCID: PMC7805417.

[11] Sabel BA, Lehnigk L. Is Mental Stress the Primary Cause of Glaucoma? Klin Monbl Augenheilkd. 2021 Feb;238(2):132–145. English, German. doi: https://doi.org/10.1055/a-1303-8025. Epub 2021 Feb 12. PMID: 33578436.

[12] Stoll, Angela. "Spiegel der Seele: Das steckt hinter Augenkrankheiten." Augsburger Allgemeine, 23 Oct. 2019, www.augsburger-allgemeine.de/wissenschaft/Sehprobleme-Spiegel-der-Seele-Das-steckt-hinter-Augenkrankheiten-id42369421.html.

Examples of psychogenic visual disorders are

- No. 17: Healing of two blind men (Mt 9:27–31).
- No. 26: Healing of the blind man of Bethsaida (Mk 8:22–26).
- No. 28: Healing of one born blind at the pool of Shiloh (Jn 9:1–7).
- No. 32: healing of the blind man at the outskirts of Jericho (Lk 18:35–43; Mk 10:46–52; Mt 20:29–34).

2.1.3 Somatoform Disorders (Psychosomatic Diseases)

In the past, somatoform disorders were referred to as psychosomatic diseases. This term was actually much more appropriate, since it already describes that mental processes can lead to physical reactions. When someone is "under pressure", high blood pressure can be the result, simply because stress is a constant emergency situation and as such increases blood pressure. Or if someone is afraid, they may "shit themselves" or "pee their pants out of fear" simply because the mental state of "fear" is coupled with the physical reaction, defecation, or urination. There are a number of such psychosomatic reactions. Most languages are full of idioms describing the connection between mental processes and physical reactions. One of the special things about psychosomatic reactions is that they can also be cured relatively quickly. A psychotherapist who recognizes the underlying conflict and is able to resolve it can sometimes achieve a very rapid healing success here. For outsiders, it may seem like a miracle how quickly someone can get better. Just as with many other mental illnesses, the prospect of salvation can often lead to healing.

In the Bible, we find several passages that can be counted among this group of illnesses. Jesus already had a tremendous reputation for healing successes. With every further success, he had an easier time. One only needs to think of all his "remote healings", where it already came to an improvement of the condition, even before he appeared himself. Merely the announcement and the prospect of healing had already led to an improvement. An example of such a miracle healing is the lowering of fever, which came about with the appearance of Jesus.

2.1.3.1 Psychogenic Fever

Why does psychogenic fever exist at all? One would think that stress does not lead to an increase in temperature. How can there be a psychosomatic reaction that leads to fever? Research has shown that infections, tumours, autoimmune diseases and predominantly inflammatory diseases lead to an increase in fever. So-called pyrogens or certain cytokines (inflammatory messengers) are required for a fever to occur.

This view is undoubtedly correct. But there are other causes of a rise in temperature. Doctors distinguish between temperature rise with chills and temperature rise without chills. The former form is the more familiar type of fever. Sufferers feel cold, although their skin may already be red-hot, and they shiver. This muscle trembling leads to a strong build up of heat and a rapid rise in temperature. That not only allows chemical defence reactions to proceed more quickly, but also allows nasty germs to be killed simply by a high temperature.

In contrast, there is the physical rise in temperature without the body and muscles shivering. Stress plays a major role in this. Especially in the abdomen ("fat belly") there is so-called brown adipose tissue. This is a special fatty tissue that is responsible for temperature regulation. The fat cells carry so-called beta-3 adrenoreceptors on their surface. This means that there is already a connection with stress. Adrenoreceptors on body cells receive signals from the stress hormones, adrenaline, and noradrenaline. Each organ has different receiving antennae, which are called adrenoreceptors. The subtypes of these adrenoreceptors are called alpha-1, alpha-2, beta-1, beta-2 and beta-3 receptors. Beta-3 receptors, which are mainly found on brown adipose tissue, are not so well known even among medical experts and are stimulated by the stress hormone adrenaline. This results in an increase in temperature due to increased fat burning, without any muscle tremors. Thus, we have the explanation why stress can lead to an increase in temperature. This also makes sense because in flight and fight behaviour everything has to go faster and with a higher temperature, biochemical reactions run faster. Depressed people who are under constant stress are also characterized by the fact that they lower their body temperature only poorly or not at all during the night. There are many more examples that could be listed here.

Stress-related or so-called psychogenic fever is sometimes also called functional hyperthermia, a rare form of fever that, as mentioned, can be triggered by psychosomatic processes such as emotional conflicts, anxiety, restlessness, or states of tension. In most cases, there is an increase in temperature to between 37.5 and 38.0 °C, rarely up to 40.0 °C. Typically, the skin and face are cool and pale, indicating increased stress hormone action. A good summary on psychogenic fever was published in 2015.[13]

There are numerous case reports in the modern literature, such as one woman who had to have both breasts removed because she had cancer. Every time the surgery was scheduled, she developed a fever, so the surgery had to be cancelled. It took a long time for the surgeons to realize that the fever could only be brought down with psychopharmaceuticals. After appropriate psychopharmacological preparation, she no longer developed a fever before the surgery date and was able to undergo surgery.[14] A case report has also been published in which someone was afraid of a COVID-19 infection and therefore spiked a fever even though he did not have an infection.[15] There are also examples in the Bible of miraculous healings from fever attributed

[13] Oka T. Psychogenic fever: how psychological stress affects body temperature in the clinical population. Temperature (Austin). 2015 Jun 3;2(3):368–78. doi: https://doi.org/10.1080/23328940.2015.1056907. PMID: 27227051; PMCID: PMC4843908.

[14] Koren SF, Engel LE, Møller MP. Preoperative psychogenic fever: to operate or not to operate. J Surg Case Rep. 2021 Mar 29;2021(3):rjab114. doi: https://doi.org/10.1093/jscr/rjab114. PMID: 33815760; PMCID: PMC8007217.

[15] Imataki O, Uemura M. Psychogenic fever due to worry about COVID-19: A case report. Clin Case Rep. 2021 Aug 16;9(8):e04560. doi: https://doi.org/10.1002/ccr3.4560. PMID: 34429986; PMCID: PMC8365391.

to the appearance of Jesus. Perhaps the first case reports of psychogenic fever or functional hyperthermia.

Examples of psychogenic fever are

- No. 5: Healing of the son of a royal official in Capernaum (Jn 4:46–54).
- No. 9: Healing of Peter's mother-in-law in Capernaum by touching her hand (Lk 4:38–39; Mk 1:29–31; Mt 8:14–15).

2.2 Diseases Mistaken for Possession (Demon Exorcisms)

Dealing with people who exhibit unusual behaviour is a problem for many people even today. When a person has an epileptic seizure, convulses, foams at the mouth and possibly even screams and falls to the ground writhing, it is really not a pleasant sight even for hard-nosed doctors. For laypersons, something like this is likely to be quite frightening.

The same applies when a schizophrenic in panic tries to flee from his own hallucinations and hides from his own inner voices and tries to bring himself to safety. If such a person possibly screams out of fear or lets these voices become loud following the "inner voices", then such an experience is also quite frightening not only for the affected person, but also for the bystanders. In addition, the voice can change dramatically during anxiety and panic. This is a generally known phenomenon, that people get a different voice pitch during fear than the one used under normal circumstances. The "tuning" changes. All these symptoms have been shown in various sensationalist Hollywood movies, where they have been associated with demons and "possession", according to the preconceptions of the layman. It is understandable that such experiences could not have been explained to people 2000 years ago. For lack of knowledge of diseases that can lead to such symptoms, such states were described as "possession".

The causes behind the descriptions of possession in the Bible are very many psychiatric and neurological illnesses that can lead to strange, uncontrolled behaviour. Among others, these are diseases such as epilepsy, schizophrenic episodes, panic attacks, hyperventilation, and outbursts of rage in the context of an intermittent explosive disorder, etc.

Excursus: Even today, official representatives of the Catholic Church still believe in possession. There are not only individual representatives of the Church who practise exorcism and devil-expelling rituals - in the Vatican News of 9.4.2018 one could read the following text: "The papal college is again offering an exorcism course: the training to become an exorcist is intended to give priests a serious scientific, theological, interdisciplinary all-round view of the subject. An exorcism is not magic, but a service of charity and mercy.

Doctors should also recognize spiritual needs. For the 13th time, a course on exorcism is being held at a papal college in Rome. The seminar, which is not open to the public, at the Regina Apostolic University from April 16 to 21 (2018), is aimed exclusively at priests who require a refresher on exorcism. Since the turn of the millennium, requests for deliverance from demons have tripled. Pedro Barrajon, a professor at the Pontifical University Regina Apostolicum, speaking to Vatican News, said the course grew out of demand from priests who felt inadequately prepared for exorcisms. The world of exorcism is not an easy terrain, said the Legionaries of Christ priest. Theology has neglected the field in recent decades, he said because it seems "out of step with the rationalist world of today". "Performing an exorcism is not a magical act", Barrajon stresses. The training, he said, seeks to provide a "serious, scientific, theological, interdisciplinary" all-around view. A priest must follow his bishop's request to serve as an exorcist, "even if he doesn't like it", Barrajon said. It is a "service of charity and mercy", he said.[16]

Overview of Bible passages in which demons or "possession" play a role

- Mt 9,32 When they had gone, behold, a mute was brought to him who was possessed by a demon (Miracle # 18).
- Mt 9:33 He cast out the demon, and the mute was able to speak. All the people were amazed and said, "Such a thing has never been seen in Israel" (Miracle #18).
- Mt 11,18 For John came, not eating and not drinking, and they say, He has a demon.
- Mt 15,22 And behold, a Canaanite woman from that region came to him and cried out: Have mercy on me, Lord, you Son of David; my daughter is tormented by a demon (Miracle #24).
- Mt 17,18 And Jesus threatened him, and the demon departed from him. And the boy was healed from that hour.
- Mt 17,19 When the disciples were alone with Jesus, they turned to Him and asked, "Why then could we not cast out the demon"?
- Mk 1,23 In their synagogue there was a man possessed by an unclean spirit.
- Mk 3,22 The scribes who had come down from Jerusalem said, "He is possessed by Beelzebul, with the help of the ruler of demons, he casts out demons".
- Mk 5,2 When he got out of the boat, immediately a man possessed by an unclean spirit ran toward him from the tombs.
- Mk 5,15 They came to Jesus and saw with Him the man who had been possessed by the legion of demons, clothed and in his right mind. Then they were afraid.
- Mk 5,18 When He got into the boat, the man who had been demon-possessed before asked Him to let him be with Him.
- Mk 7,25 A woman whose daughter was possessed by an unclean spirit heard about Him; she immediately came and fell at His feet.

[16] https://www.vaticannews.va/de/vatikan/news/2018-04/exorzismus-teufelsaustreibung-paepstliche-universitaet.html, accessed 8.8.2019.

- Mk 7,26 The woman, a Syro-Phoenician by birth, was a Gentile. She asked him to cast out the demon from her daughter.
- Mk 7,29 He answered her, "Because you have said this, I say to you, go home"; the demon has left your daughter.
- Mk 7,30 And when she came home, she found the child lying on the bed and saw that the demon had left her.
- Mk 9,17 One of the crowd answered him, "Teacher, I have brought my son to you. He is possessed by a dumb spirit".
- Mk 9:28 Jesus entered the house, and his disciples, when they were alone, asked him: Why then could we not cast out the demon?
- Lk 4:33 There was a man in the synagogue who was possessed by a demon, an unclean spirit. He cried out with a loud voice
- Lk 4,35 Then Jesus threatened him, "Be silent and leave him". The demon threw the man into their midst and left him without harming him.
- Lk 7,33 For John the Baptist has come, eating no bread and drinking no wine, and you say, He has a demon.
- Lk 8,27 When Jesus went ashore, a man from the city who was demon-possessed ran to meet Him. For a long time, he had not worn any clothes and had not lived in a house but in the caves of the grave.
- Lk 8,29 Jesus had in fact commanded the unclean spirit to leave the man. For a long time, the spirit had held him in its power, and he was bound with chains and shackles and held captive. But again and again he broke the fetters and was driven by the demon into deserted places.
- Lk 8,30 Jesus asked him: What is your name? He answered, Legion. For he was possessed by many demons.
- Lk 9,42 When the son came here, the demon threw him to the ground and dragged him to and fro. But Jesus threatened the unclean spirit, healed the boy and returned him to his father.
- Lk 11:14 Jesus cast out a demon that was mute. And it came to pass that when the demon was cast out, the man was able to speak. All the people were amazed.
- John 7:20 The crowd answered, "You are possessed by a demon. Who then is seeking to kill you"?
- John 8,48 Then the Jews answered Him, "Do we not rightly say, 'You are a Samaritan and possessed by a demon"?
- John 8:49 Jesus replied: I am not possessed by a demon, but I honour my Father; but you revile me.
- John 8,52 Then the Jews said to Him, "Now we know that You are possessed by a demon. Abraham and the prophets died, but you say, If anyone holds fast to my word, he will not suffer death forever".
- John 10:20 Many of them said, He is demon-possessed and speaks in delusion. Why do you listen to him?
- John 10,21 Others said, "No possessed person talks like that. Can a demon open the eyes of the blind"?

2.2.1 Intermittent Explosive Disorder

Anger outbursts are usually an expression of a psychiatric disorder, are accompanied by changes in personality and can be quite frightening. One of the most common causes of anger outbursts is *intermittent explosive disorder.*

Intermittent explosive disorder is defined as "repeated failure to resist aggressive impulses". The impulses can also lead to severe violence, destruction of property, and mental violence. In common parlance, such people are described as "freaks" or "irascible" or, in their mildest form, simply as "irritable" or as "short-tempered". In any case, a pronounced loss of impulse control can be very frightening for those nearby.

In the absence, of modern psychiatric knowledge, one can imagine that such people used to be considered "possessed by demons". As the episodes of an outburst of anger are limited in time, people appear afterwards "as if freed from a demon". Such outbursts of anger are very stressful, not only for bystanders, but also for the affected person. They are usually sorry after such an attack and would like to undo everything if it were possible. Often they also apologize, but unfortunately this is no guarantee that there will not be another outburst of rage on the next occasion.

Intermittent explosive disorder can be distinguished from the "choleric" character in that affected persons show a kind of remorse after an attack and are sorry for everything. In personality disorders that involve outbursts of anger (choleric), the affected person usually does not feel bad after a rage, but feels that his or her explosive behaviour is "justified". Nowadays, both impulse control loss and personality disorder belong in the hands of a psychiatrist or psychotherapist. They require behaviour therapy and frequently also drug therapy, especially since disturbances in serotonin metabolism play a role here. With children, it is different. Here, outbursts of rage can occur as a "normal" phenomenon in the course of development. However, if they persist into adulthood, they have the character of a disease.

Examples of demon exorcisms in the NT (Mark's Gospel in particular reports numerous exorcisms)

- No. 8: The possessed man in the synagogue of Capernaum (Mk 1:21–28).
- No. 19: Healing of the possessed man from Gerasa (Mk 5:1–20; Mt 8:28–34; Lk 8:26–39).

2.2.2 Panic Attacks and Hyperventilation Syndrome

The most impressive healing successes can be experienced with panic attacks that are accompanied by hyperventilation syndrome. Sufferers offer a rather dramatic performance to those around them. People present frequently believe that the affected person will die right now if competent help does not come immediately. For people present who have to witness something like this, the situation is almost always an extraordinary burden, especially since no one knows how to react. If such a hyperventilation syndrome lasts for a longer period of time, the fear is often transferred to the bystanders. This creates a social interaction in which not only the panic attack is worsened in the first person affected. It can even happen that other people react as well and also develop panic attacks. For example, the mother may herself develop a panic attack with hyperventilation tetany in response to her daughter's panic attack. When medical help arrives, several people then have to be treated.

In the context of a hyperventilation syndrome, people often start screaming and thus put people in fear and terror. In such situations, bystanders usually react with pronounced helplessness. This, in turn, increases the fear of those affected even more because they realize that no one can help them. Sometimes groups of people can get into a panic reaction and behave very strangely. When whole groups are affected, this can take on quite dramatic proportions and lead to mass panic or mass psychosis.

Recovery from hyperventilation syndrome occurs at the latest when the affected person becomes unconscious. The anxiety then subsides, breathing levels off again, the pH value in the blood returns to normal and the nerves resume their normal function. Such "healing processes" can be accelerated if someone comes and radiates calmness or sovereignty. Someone who lays on a hand or gives orders and thus distracts the patient from the exciting situation. In today's clinical routine, the appearance of the doctor is often enough for the whole affair to calm down again. From this viewpoint, a doctor can work "miracles" merely by appearing. The mere prospect of healing can bring about actual healing. The well-known physician Balint also spoke of the "drug doctor" in such cases.

Bible passages in which hyperventilation could have played a role

- No. 12: The healing of a paralytic (Luke 5:17–26).
- No. 13: Sabbath, healing (Luke 6:6–10).
- No. 20: The raising of a synagogue ruler's daughter and the healing of a sick woman (Luke 8:41–56).
- No. 23: The revelation of the Son of God on the water (Mark 6:45–52; Matthew 14:22–33; John 6:16–21).

2.2.3 Epileptic and Psychogenic Non-epileptic Seizures (PNES)

Epilepsy is a collective name for a group of brain dysfunctions caused by uncontrolled excitation of nerves and lack of inhibition of excitation propagation in the brain". This is the somewhat awkward-sounding definition of an entire group of diseases. Seen from the outside, epilepsy can take very different forms. On the one hand, there are generalized seizures in which the affected person falls to the ground ("falling sickness"), convulses, possibly lets out a scream and foams at the mouth, and then falls into a twilight state. Such seizures are quite dramatic and unpleasant experiences for bystanders present.

On the other hand, epileptic seizures can go completely unnoticed by others. For example, children may appear only temporarily "mentally absent" or may simply be seen by their teachers as "inattentive students" because they have recurrent mental absences. In another case of epilepsy, there are only involuntary muscle movements of individual muscle groups (myoclonus, focal motor seizures). Alternatively, nothing is seen from the outside and the affected person experiences "only" hallucinations, possibly only a feeling of pressure in the abdomen or ants running down the arm (focal sensory seizures). Such seizures, which are often difficult to distinguish from a schizophrenic episode, are also called "aura". Or a seizure may manifest merely as a "Déjà vu experience". Sometimes there are also changes in emotional experience. In addition, epileptic disorders frequently occur in combination with psychiatric disorders. Such psychic abnormalities are also called "alternative psychosis".

The doctors in ancient times already knew about this disease and called it the disease of the saints or "morbus sacer", probably because people affected by epilepsy had visions and had "contact with gods". Caesar was one of the most famous people in ancient times who suffered from "morbus sacer". Conversely, affected people have been considered "possessed" because of their recurrent inexplicable behaviour. Sometimes such people have been locked away from society, probably because they were feared. In any case, epileptic seizures can lead to a series of events that may be perceived by others as "inexplicable". The public then speaks of "peculiar" behaviour, "obsession", "being odd", or simply of a "weirdo". Epileptic seizures are not that rare: About 2–4% of all people experience a single, isolated epileptic seizure in their lifetime, and about 0.5–1% develop epilepsy.

Psychogenic seizures must be distinguished from true epilepsy. Today they are called "psychogenic non-epileptic seizures (PNES)" and are classified as dissociative disorders. In former times this group of diseases was called neuroses or more precisely conversion neuroses. Even earlier, one spoke of hysteria. In principle, however, they are all the same and only interpreted differently in the course of history and therefore called differently. Dissociative seizures (PNES) bear a strong resemblance to epileptic seizures. However, there are significant differences. For example, there are never symptoms typical of epilepsy, such as tongue biting, fall injuries, or defecation and urination. In addition, the affected person is not completely unconscious during the seizure, but may enter a trance-like state. The pattern of seizures also appears different. There are convulsive twitches, contortions, hyperextension of the head, grimacing or shaking movements of the arms, legs, or head. After a seizure, there is only fragmentary or no memory of the seizure. The incidence of such dissociative seizures is low, occurring in about 20–23 people per 100,000 population. Women are more often affected than men, which may be due to the fact that hormonal cycles can lead to a change in respiration and thus in nerve function. Accordingly, the first seizures usually occur at the onset of puberty. The causes of such psychogenic non-epileptic seizures are not really known. However, many affected individuals have experienced trauma. The trauma may have occurred a very long time ago and is frequently not remembered. During a seizure, however, flashbacks may occur with re-experiencing of the trauma either during the day or at night as a nightmare. Very difficult life situations are also possible causes of dissociative seizures. Especially unusually strong and seemingly hopeless conflicts in the family or at work should be mentioned here. The treatment of such seizures (PNES) today consists of psychotherapy. As first aid for such situations, it is recommended today to provide a "safe atmosphere" and to talk calmly and kindly with the affected person.

In the Bible, it is striking that Jesus repeatedly took his "patients" aside to talk to them in peace, away from other people. This alone may have miraculously healed many a dissociative disorder.

Concomitant diseases of PNES: 90% of the affected persons have concomitant mental diseases. The most common comorbidities include:

- Other dissociative disorders,
- Somatoform disorders,
- Depression,
- Anxiety disorders,
- Personality disorders,
- Post-traumatic stress disorders.

2.2.4 *Schizophrenia, Perceptual Disorders, Hallucinogens (Entheogens)*

Perceptual disorders such as hallucinations are among the leading symptoms of schizophrenic psychoses. Since perceptual disorders have been encountered continuously in the Bible since Adam and Eve, and since there are different forms of perceptual disorders, they will be discussed in more detail here.

2.2.4.1 Types of Perceptual Disorders

Most people believe they are free from perceptual disorders. However, we do not all perceive the world as it really is. Rather, the world is seen in such a way that our perception gives us a good chance of survival. This leads us, for example, to overestimate heights and depths, while lengths and widths are relatively correctly estimated. This misjudgment saves us from jumping into "dangerous" depths. It may not correspond to reality, but it increases our probability of remaining unharmed. In this sense, we all have a "wrong" perception, so to speak. On top of that, perceptions have to be interpreted. Things we see, hear, or smell must first be compared to empirical values before they can be interpreted and named. Errors often occur in the process. Errors in the detection of events in the environment are called perceptual disorders. The transition from "normally disturbed" perception to "pathologically disturbed" perception is fluid.

Here's an example: Imagine you are driving a car along a wooded road in winter. Dusk is falling. The lighting conditions are poor, and you can see something moving in the distance. You slow down because you think you recognize a person in the moving figure. Only when you get closer do you realize that it is not a person, but an animal. Psychiatrists refer to this form of sensory illusion as "illusory misperception". The essential characteristic of illusory misperception or illusion is that an object is present but is misinterpreted.

In contrast, there is the more pronounced form of a perceptual disorder in which one sees or hears something even though nothing is present. In other words, a triggering sensory stimulus is missing. Physicians speak in such a case of hallucinations. Then there are so-called pseudo-hallucinations, in which, as in the case of a real hallucination, something is perceived without a triggering stimulus, but the person concerned is aware that it is a mirage and not a real object. Thus, there is hallucination insight. In real hallucinations, there is no insight of a hallucination.

In the Bible, the story is told of Moses seeing a burning thorn bush. If this was a thorn bush moving in the wind, then it would be an illusory misperception. If a burning thorn bush were seen that was not there at all, that would be a hallucination. From the example of the Bible, we cannot recognize today whether it may have been an illusory misperception or a hallucination in the case of Moses. One can only exclude a pseudo-hallucination, since the further history of Moses does not point to any hallucination insight.

Another escalation of hallucination is when one not only hears voices, but also begins to speak with them. Or when these voices give commands. This form of hallucinations is called "dialogizing voices" or "imperative voices" by psychiatrists, and they are already considered as first degree symptoms for the diagnosis of schizophrenia. In the Bible, there are numerous examples of God or an angel talking to someone and giving orders. This is a symptom that already strongly suggests the presence of a psychosis of the schizophrenic form.

Perceptual disorders can affect not only the sense of hearing and sight, but all other senses. Thus also smell sensations can occur, which have no actual source or are felt "wrongly". Fragrant scents can be perceived as smelly or, conversely, stench can be perceived as fragrant. Or one smells something, although others perceive no odour. Tactile stimuli are perceived as particularly unpleasant when one feels "touched" although no one is there or the stimulus was merely triggered by a breeze. How often such a thing occurs can also be seen in the language used when one feels "pleasantly or unpleasantly touched" by an occurrence. Sometimes persons feel wetness on their skin, although it is not there, etc.

Abnormal sensations of taste can also occur. Metal tastes may be an initial symptom of the onset of schizophrenia. Or a taste that you can't get rid of. Any sense can be affected, and each perceptual disturbance can have varying degrees of severity. However, auditory hallucinations (hearing voices) and visual hallucinations (seeing things that are not there) are most common. An overview of perceptual disorders is given in the table below.

Quantitative Differences of Perceptual Disorders

- Illusory misperception (object is present but is misinterpreted, E.g. "Floating log is interpreted as Jesus walking on water").
- Hallucination (no object is present, but one sees, hears, smells or feels something. The person affected does NOT realize that these are mirages. E.g. "Appearance of angels speaking to one").
- Pseudohallucinations are hallucinations, but the affected person recognizes that it must be a perceptual disorder. There is hallucination insight. (E.g. "I see people who look like trees").

Qualitative Differences Among Perceptual Disorders

- optical hallucinations (objects are seen, "apparitions")
- auditory hallucinations (people talk to or about you)
- olfactory hallucinations (special scents are smelled)
- gustatory hallucinations (gustatory sensations, e.g., metallic taste)
- haptic hallucinations (one feels touched, attacked)

2.2.4.2 Factors Favouring Perceptual Disturbances

The occurrence of hallucinations seems to have a congenital component on the one hand, but on the other hand there are also external circumstances, so-called triggers, which can trigger hallucinations.

Genetic Predisposition

Schizophrenia and the tendency to perceptual disorders run in families. Therefore, a genetic cause has long been suspected. Only recently have the corresponding genes also been discovered and published. See also table below.

More and more publications are appearing that point to a genetic predisposition for schizophrenia. As of 2014, 108 schizophrenia-associated gene loci have been described.[17] These include alterations in the following genes: DOCK4, CEACAM21, PGBD1, RELN,

---

[17] Schizophrenia Working Group of the Psychiatric Genomics Consortium (2014). Biological insights from 108 schizophrenia-associated genetic loci. Nature, 511(7510), 421–427. https://doi.org/10.1038/nature13595 .

PRODH,[18] CACNA1C,[19] PCDHA3,[20] NDST3,[21] hKCa3/KCNN3.[22] Today, the lifetime prevalence, i.e., the probability of developing schizophrenia throughout life, is reported to be 1–2%[23] or the incidence to be 0.11–0.7 per 1000 population per year.[24] This means that something like one in 50–100 people will experience a schizophrenic episode once in their lifetime. In addition, there is an up to tenfold increased occurrence of schizophrenic episodes after migration.[25] However, this increased risk is attributed by some authors to psychosocial stress rather than genetic factors.[26] Since the incidence in poor countries of the Third World is about twice as high as in rich countries,[27] one may assume that also in biblical times the incidence of psychoses was probably twice as high as in modern times.

The genetic predisposition for hallucinations is perhaps also significant in the Bible. In the Old Testament, from Adam and Eve in paradise to Noah, Abraham, Moses, etc., there is repeated mention of "visions" and commands from God (imperative voices) and conversations with God (dialogizing voices). It is interesting that in

---

[18] Alkelai, Anna, et al. "DOCK4 and CEACAM21 as novel schizophrenia candidate genes in the Jewish population." Int. J. Neuropsychopharmacol., vol. 15, no. 4, May. 2012, pp. 459–69, doi: https://doi.org/10.1017/S1461145711000903.

[19] Wang, Zuxing, et al. "An independent, replicable, functional and significant risk variant block at intron 3 of CACNA1C for schizophrenia." Aust. N. Z. J. Psychiatry, vol. 48674211009595., 2 May. 2021, doi: https://doi.org/10.1177/00048674211009595.

[20] Lencz, Todd, et al. "Novel ultra-rare exonic variants identified in a founder population implicate cadherins in schizophrenia." Neuron, vol. 109, no. 9, 5 May. 2021, pp. 1465–14784, doi: https://doi.org/10.1016/j.neuron.2021.03.004.

[21] Lencz, Todd, et al. "Genome-wide association study implicates NDST3 in schizophrenia and bipolar disorder." Nat. Commun., vol. 4, no. 2739, 19 Nov. 2013, pp. 1–10, doi: https://doi.org/10.1038/ncomms3739.

[22] Dror, V., et al. "hKCa3/KCNN3 potassium channel gene: association of longer CAG repeats with schizophrenia in Israeli Ashkenazi Jews, expression in human tissues and localization to chromosome 1q21." Mol. Psychiatry, vol. 4, May. 1999, pp. 254–60, doi: https://doi.org/10.1038/sj.mp.4000508.

[23] DocCheck Medical Services GmbH. "Schizophrenie—DocCheck Flexikon." DocCheck Flexikon, 27 Apr. 2021, https://flexikon.doccheck.com/de/Schizophrenie.

[24] Messias, E. L., Chen, C. Y., & Eaton, W. W. (2007). Epidemiology of schizophrenia: review of findings and myths. The Psychiatric clinics of North America, 30(3), 323–338. https://doi.org/10.1016/j.psc.2007.04.007 .

[25] Eaton W, Harrison G. Ethnic disadvantage and schizophrenia. Acta Psychiatr Scand Suppl. 2000;(407):38–43. doi: https://doi.org/10.1034/j.1600-0447.2000.00007.x. PMID: 11261638.

[26] Messias, E. L., Chen, C. Y., & Eaton, W. W. (2007). Epidemiology of schizophrenia: review of findings and myths. The Psychiatric clinics of North America, 30(3), 323–338. https://doi.org/10.1016/j.psc.2007.04.007.

[27] Cohen A. Prognosis for schizophrenia in the Third World: a reevaluation of cross-cultural research. Cult Med Psychiatry. 1992 Mar;16(1):53–75; discussion 77–106. doi: https://doi.org/10.1007/BF00054439. PMID: 1537236.

the Bible the kinship between the biblical patriarchs and the descent with enumeration of the family members is indicated quite exactly. Again and again schizoid traits are found in all generations of which stories are told in the Bible. Also, Christ as "son of David" (Mt 1,20), was probably subject to this genetic predisposition, which makes it understandable that he also experienced dialogizing voices.

If perceptual disorders are so common, they must also hold advantages from an evolutionary perspective. It is important to realize that perceptual disorders have nothing to do with intelligence or other brain performance. Affected individuals can be extremely intelligent, demonstrate high mental performance, and readily assume leadership positions. Perceptual disorders can even have advantages: artists can use them to fire their imagination, technicians can come up with more creative inventions, and scientists can develop unorthodox ideas and thus be at the forefront. These are all qualities that drive the development of a society.

The higher the social position of a person with disturbed perception, the more he has to justify it by confabulations[28] (rationalization in the psychological sense). This gives rise to "unbelievable" attempts at explanation and interpretations such as "God himself has spoken to me". With children one can often see with which fantasy and how excitedly they embellish (confabulate) what they have experienced, not in order to lie to their parents, but simply so that what they have experienced fits into "their" world view. We are inclined to tell the children that they should not lie, but in their world and at that moment the story told is absolutely real for them. In the same way, one can imagine that it was "real" for a prince or patriarch in biblical times when "God spoke".

Triggers of Hallucinations

In addition to genetic predisposition, there are also external circumstances that can lead to perceptual disturbances., or that a relapse occurs in the context of a schizophrenic illness. These include craniocerebral trauma, infections, hunger, thirst, ingestion of drugs, alcohol, medications, or (food) toxins, as well as all life circumstances that are associated with increased stress. Thus, anxiety, panic, and hyperventilation can also lead to perceptual disturbances. But also isolation-stress, i.e. the lack of environmental stimuli, can lead to perceptual disturbances. When Jesus went into the desert and experienced hunger, thirst, stimulus deprivation, and possibly fear, one can well imagine that this situation triggered hallucinations and dialoguing voices with the devil (Matthew 4:1–11). In other places in the Bible, fear (Matthew 14:22–230), hunger, thirst, and lack of stimulation (Mark 1:12–13) are the most common triggers for hallucinations. The most common triggers of hallucinations will be discussed in more detail. However, stimulation stress, i.e. the lack of environmental stimuli, can also lead to perceptual disturbances.

---

[28] Autoren der Wikimedia-Projekte. "Konfabulation – Wikipedia." 9 Apr. 2004, https://de.wikipedia.org/w/index.php?title=Konfabulation&oldid=215924122.

Perceptual disorders are so common that probably everyone has been affected by them. Thus, one may argue whether dreaming is not a form of perceptual disorder. However, since (almost) everyone dreams, it is considered "normal". Nevertheless, dreams do not represent a real image of the environment. During the transition from the dream state to the waking state, the risk of perceptual disorders increases. Thus, some people have difficulty switching from the dream world to the real world and have states in which they cannot completely separate dream and reality. If these states occur when waking up, they are called hypnagogic states or, conversely, hypnopompic states when falling asleep. Some people can daydream. This goes so far that things that are present are interpreted differently (illusions), or that non-existent things are seen (hallucinations).

Anxiety

Hallucinations can cause anxiety and, conversely, anxiety can also cause hallucinations. This can cause the sufferer to enter a vicious cycle and remain trapped in the hallucination. An example in the Bible of this would be the apostles travelling across the Sea of Galilee, experiencing a threatening storm, and then becoming afraid. Fear predestines to trigger hallucinations in such a case. If, on top of that, visibility is poor due to the storm, and fish toxins from a previous meal may be impairing brain function, it is easy to imagine hallucinations occurring (Mk 6:45–52; Mt 14:22–33; John 6:16–21, miracle #23). Once anxiety has triggered hallucinations, and if the hallucinations are so threatening to the affected individuals that they intensify the anxiety, they can keep the affected individuals "trapped" in the hallucination. In this way, complex experiences can be explained.

Hunger and Thirst

Any form of disturbance in the water or electrolyte balance can on the one hand trigger epileptic seizures, which are often preceded by an aura with sensory illusions, or lead to disturbances in perception such as hallucinations. Since thirst can last for a long time, hallucinations triggered by thirst can also last for a long time. So, when Jesus goes into the desert and fasts there for 40 days and presumably also thirsts, delusions, and hallucinations can occur here merely from the liquid deprivation. In addition, there was also stimulus poverty, which for its part can also lead to hallucinations. So one can well imagine that Jesus had "dialogues" with the devil in the desert in this way (Mk 1,13). Something similar may have been the case with Moses, who withdrew to Mount Sinai for a long time "to speak with God".

Stimuli Deprivation

Stimulus deprivation can trigger hallucinations. Prisoners in solitary confinement therefore often have hallucinations. In principle, hallucinations can be induced in (almost) anyone if they are shielded from external environmental stimuli for long enough. Darkroom delirium is what this is called in medical parlance. Shepherds, who do not have much to do and are exposed to few stimuli, have a high incidence of this. In Westphalia, they are therefore called “Spökenkieker” (“ghost-seers”) because they repeatedly have visions. People who got lost in the desert and were then saved frequently report hallucinatory experiences. This is probably what happened to Jesus in the desert and to Moses at Mount Sinai. Another example is blind people who suddenly regain “sight” by having visual hallucinations. This phenomenon is also known as “phantom vision” and has been described several times.

Hallucinogens and Entheogens

Another trigger for hallucinations is the ingestion of substances that regularly cause perceptual disturbances. Such substances are called hallucinogens. Hallucinogens that are taken as part of cultic acts to “expand consciousness” are also called entheogens. Entheogens have been used in ritual acts for thousands of years and have been used in almost all cultures.

Triggering Causes (Triggers) of Perceptual Disorders (Selection)

- Extreme situations (stress)
  - Thirst
  - Hunger
  - Fear
  - Stages of grief
- Under-challenge stress
  - Lack of stimulation (solitary confinement, staying in the desert or in lonely places)
  - Meditation
- Drugs
  - Hallucinogens
  - Entheogens
- Brain organic disorders
  - Senile dementia, Lewy body dementia
  - Brain tumours
  - Liver or kidney failure
  - Alcohol disease
  - Cerebral hypoxia
  - Fever
- Transitional phase from sleep to wakefulness.
  - Hypnagogic states

- Hypnopompic states
- Neuropsychiatric diseases.
  - Schizophrenia, schizoaffective disorders, and other diseases of the schizophrenic type
  - Post-traumatic stress disorder (PTSD)
  - Anxiety disorder
  - Developmental disorders
  - Epilepsy.

Special attention will be paid to hallucinogenic drugs, especially since they are used in almost all religions and are referred to as "entheogens" in this function. They are used in religious acts to facilitate or intensify the experience of God. For example, people who have ingested such substances report "feeling 'one' with the universe". Many entheogens are not only "mind-expanding", but also have an antidepressant and anxiety-relieving effect that can last for weeks to months after the acute effect has worn off. Perhaps this was also a reason why priests at all times and in many cultures have often used these substances.

Entheogens include, for example, various psychoactive mushrooms such as the plant decoction "Ayahuasca" or the Aztec sage (Salvia divinorum). These are used by indigenous cultures in South and Central America and the Caribbean. In the Rastafarian faith, which originated in Jamaica, cannabis (ganja) is used as an intoxicant in a ritualistic manner. In the Indian religion of Shivaism, there is a long tradition of using hashish (charas): Indian ascetic "holy men" (sadhus) sometimes smoke their local chillum pipes daily. The traditional hemp preparation (bhang) is also used in religious rituals. Already in the Rigveda, the oldest part of the Vedic scriptures, Soma is mentioned, a sap of a plant mixed with (sour) milk as a ritual drink for sacrifices as well as an intoxicating drink of the gods. In the Christian Jewish religions, incense is still used today, which in low concentrations has an anxiety-relieving effect, but in higher concentrations can have a hallucinatory effect. This effect can be caused by the incensole contained in frankincense, which affects so-called TRPV3 channels in the neurons of the brain.[29] Thus, when incense is used in churches, the people who get only low concentrations experience a "pleasant, anxiety-relieving" effect, while the priest who gets higher concentrations may experience an "entheogenic, mind-expanding" effect.

There are repeated references to "smoke offerings" in the Bible. Unfortunately, it is not specified there which substances were used. However, one can assume that the substances used, as in most other cultures, had mind-expanding, entheogenic effects.

---

[29] Moussaieff A, Rimmerman N, Bregman T, Straiker A, Felder CC, Shoham S, Kashman Y, Huang SM, Lee H, Shohami E, Mackie K, Caterina MJ, Walker JM, Fride E, Mechoulam R. Incensole acetate, an incense component, elicits psychoactivity by activating TRPV3 channels in the brain. FASEB J. 2008 Aug;22(8):3024–34. doi: https://doi.org/10.1096/fj.07-101865. Epub 2008 May 20. PMID: 18492727; PMCID: PMC2493463.

In any case, the story of Zechariah, in the context of his smoke offering, may have been hallucinatory experiences. This is supported by the appearance of angels with whom he could converse in the form of "dialogizing voices".

Hallucinogens (Entheogens) Used for Ritual Acts

- Egyptian henbane: nightshade plant.
- Farmer's tobacco: nightshade plant.
- Angel's trumpet: Nightshade plant.
- Fly agaric: intoxicant among Siberian peoples.
- Mandrake: used as a "magic plant".
- Common or white datura: hallucinogen used in Central Europe.
- Sky-blue showy vine: a climbing plant from Mexico.
- Kava: intoxicating pepper.
- Black belladonna: Atropa belladonna.
- Black henbane: witchweed.
- Dream herb: Aztec dream grass.
- Frankincense: Resin of Boswellia trees, found in the Near East and India, used in Egypt.
- DMT (Dimethyltryptamine) natural occurrence in
  - Banisteriopsis caapi (tropical liana species)
  - Phalaris arundinacea (reed canary grass)
  - Mimosa hostilis
  - Codariocalyx motorius (telegraph plant)
  - Numerous representatives of the genus Acacia
  - Skin secretion of the Aga toad
    See also "The sacred mushroom and the cross".[30]

Warning: Many of the substances mentioned have serious harmful effects on some people, and several have therefore been banned by governments.

Miracles in which perceptual disturbances may have played a role

- No. 2: The announcement of the birth of John the Baptist, the story of Zechariah (Lk 1:5–25).
- No. 3: The miracle of the virgin birth (Lk 1:26–38 and Mt 1:18–25).
- No. 23: Jesus walking on water (Mk 6:45–52; Mt 14:22–33; Jn 6:16–21).

[30] John M. Allegro's book: The sacred mushroom and the cross (1970).

2.3 Raising from the Dead

When the dead are raised, the first thought that comes to mind is that it really must have been a miracle. As a physician, however, the first thing that comes to mind is that these may not have been real deaths, but apparent deaths, and that the original determination of death was not correct.

Most people believe that it is relatively easy to determine death. However, even for doctors in our time, it is not a simple matter to determine death quite correctly, especially if it is a recently deceased person without certain signs of death. If a corpse is decomposed or only the bones are left, the matter is clear: the person is dead. But what about when the body has not yet decomposed? When the body is still warm? If the body even appears to be or is still perfused with blood? It is little known that the brain can be really dead while the heart is still beating (brain death without circulatory death). Conversely, the heart can stop beating without brain death having occurred at the same time (circulatory death without brain death). The whole of transplantation surgery would not be possible without the distinction between cardiac death and brain death because the donor organs must be removed while the heart is still beating, otherwise they would not be usable at all.

2.3.1 *How Death Is Determined Nowadays*

The pathologist, who has to be sure that the body is a corpse before he opens it during the autopsy, distinguishes between certain and uncertain signs of death. Death marks, for example, are a certain sign of death, but even the determination of death marks is not easy for a layman. I can still remember how a medical student got into distress because he was not sure whether the stains on a corpse were already certain death marks or only stains in the context of hypostasis. And whether the stains could be pushed away or not, as that would be an essential characteristic for whether they were real death marks or not. The medical student in question passed his pathology examination at that time, but was in real distress.

In daily life, knowing the sure signs of death is irrelevant. As an average person, one will hardly face the embarrassment of having to determine death. A doctor who has to issue a death certificate, however, will have to deal more with the determination of certain death. Therefore, doctors do not only examine whether consciousness has been lost. They also examine whether reflexes are absent, whether there is no response to pain stimuli, whether the pulse is still palpable, whether breathing has stopped, and so on. But all these are only uncertain signs of death. That is why doctors also avail themselves of the help of diagnostic equipment to determine death. They record an ECG to deduce the electrical currents of the heart. A zero line in the ECG already speaks very much for death having occurred. But even here there are uncertainties, and it depends on how long the zero line has existed. A few minutes can pass and there is still a possibility of resuscitation. For this reason, the more reliable method has recently been adopted, namely to write an EEG report by recording the brain waves. If a zero line is found here, the patient is called brain-dead, which is inevitably followed by the death of the entire body.

Especially for the removal of organs for transplantation purposes, the EEG, and brain death are used to get the "permission" to remove organs. But even here there are incidents where, for example, a medical technical assistant has received blood from a brain-dead patient for the planned organ removal in order to perform the appropriate HLA typings necessary for the transplantation. While she was in the middle of the typing, she received a call from the transplant surgeon, and was able to stop the (complex) HLA examination because, the (dead) patient had "woken up" and regained consciousness. Such experiences may have occurred more often, which is why today the repeated zero line in the EEG at an interval of at least 30 min is mandatory before organs can be removed.

The rules for this differ in Austria, Germany, and Switzerland. Are there regional differences here as to when a person is dead? How ambiguous the guidelines for death determination are, can also be seen from the fact that the joint statements of various German medical societies on death determination were reissued in 1994, 1997, 2011, 2002, 2012, 2014, 2015, and 2016 respectively.[31] One would think that the process of dying does not change. Apparently, however, even doctors don't quite agree on when someone is dead. If you download the article on brain death on Wikipedia, you get a whole 21 pages, and then afterwards you still don't know exactly how best to define death. Doctors, lawyers, and theologians apparently use different definitions here and each speaks a different language.

One must therefore conclude that the definition of death is an arbitrary one. When is the human being dead? When his last cell has died and can no longer reproduce? And what about DNA, which can be extracted from mummies even after thousands of years? But even if one uses common sense to define death, there are still macabre stories about the determination of death in the community. For example, there is a rumour among doctors that a patient with barbiturate poisoning was found to be dead by a doctor. When the "corpse" arrived at the coroner's office, it was still successfully resuscitated by the coroners in the autopsy room. Whether this rumour is true or not, I do not know. Nor is it significant. The story is only to illustrate that the determination of death is really not easy. Even among experts and with the aid of modern diagnostic equipment, there are still problems in determining death. What is meant to be said with this illustration is that it can be assumed that death really could not be determined correctly 2000 years ago.

---

[31] Buchner H, Ferbert A. Irreversibilitätsnachweis der klinischen Ausfallssymptome des Gehirns. Elektroenzephalographie und evozierte Potenziale [Determination of irreversibility of clinical brain death. Electroencephalography and evoked potentials]. Nervenarzt. 2016 Feb;87(2):128–42. German. doi: https://doi.org/10.1007/s00115-015-0049-x. PMID: 26785843.

2.3.2 "Vita Minima" or Apparent Death

In the case of the miracles described in the Bible involving resurrection from the dead (Christ after crucifixion) or the resurrection to life (the story of Lazarus), it is very questionable whether people were really dead. If it is hardly possible for experts today to determine death with absolute certainty, it is very unlikely that people in ancient times could determine death with real certainty. At that time, the most one could do was to check consciousness, pulse or breathing, all signs that are absolutely incapable of determining death.

Most readers will have seen an unconscious person at some point in their lives. The most common is to see people who have collapsed, are unconscious on the floor for a short time, and then are able to get up again (syncope). It is rarer to have seen an unconscious person whose pulse could no longer be reliably felt and whose breathing could no longer be perceived (e.g. in shock). Such persons are usually immediately taken to the hospital by ambulance for treatment. Yes, even with calmly sleeping people, it is not always sure whether they are still breathing. So, it often happens that such sleeping people are shaken awake to make sure that they are still alive.

Until recently, the term "vita minima" was used in medical terminology. This term was used to describe a condition in which a person was unconscious, the pulse was no longer palpable and breathing was no longer perceptible. Only with appropriate medical monitoring equipment could it be seen that the heartbeat and breathing were still present. When people can no longer detect signs of life, as is the case with the term vita minima, the term apparent death is used in common parlance. The term "apparent death" was first used by the physician Dr. J. G. Krünitz in 1788.[32] Before that, people were apparently not even aware that there can be a state similar to death, but where death has not actually occurred. Today, most cultures and languages have terms such as "suspended animation".

The way of death ascertainment, as it was practised in antiquity, appears downright ridiculous. It was usual to call the dead person several times by name and then declare death if he did not answer.[33] With such a way of establishing death, one can assume that there were at that time very many humans, who were wrongly presumed to be dead and were buried alive.

Apparently, this was also suspected in the past. Especially in the Age of Enlightenment from the seventeenth century to the nineteenth century, there was great fear in Europe of being buried alive.[34] Therefore, people were given a "death bell" in the coffin. With it, the dead should be able to make themselves noticeable, if actually still alive. The laying out of the dead may also have been justified by this because the fear of being buried alive always accompanied people.

[32] Autoren der Wikimedia-Projekte. "Scheintod – Wikipedia." 14 Sept. 2004, https://de.wikipedia.org/w/index.php?title=Scheintod&oldid=217070636.

[33] "Die Todesfeststellung in der Geschichte der Medizin." MTA Dialog, 22 Nov. 2021, www.mta-dialog.de/artikel/die-todesfeststellung-in-der-geschichte-der-medizin.html.

[34] Autoren der Wikimedia-Projekte. "Scheintod – Wikipedia." 14 Sept. 2004, https://de.wikipedia.org/w/index.php?title=Scheintod&oldid=217070636.

In the Mediterranean countries, it was and still is customary to bury a dead person quickly. Thus, even today in some countries, dead bodies must be buried within 24 h. Under such circumstances, a reliable determination of death cannot actually be made for all corpses. Under such customs or even legal regulations, one must assume that also in our time in some countries people were and still are buried alive. So, it must have been with the young man of Naïn (Luke 7:11–17). He was hastily carried out of the city to be buried. Jesus went to the bier and apparently had enough time to look at the presumed dead man, observe his breathing and possibly feel for a pulse. As was the custom at the time to determine death, he called him and gave him the order to get up. With success, as the story describes.

Raising the dead in the New Testament

- No. 1: crucifixion and resurrection of Jesus Christ (Lk 23:26–49; Mk 15:20–28; Mt 27:31–62, Jn 19:1–42).
- No. 15: Raising of the young man of Naïn (Lk 7:11–17).
- No. 20: daughter of Jaïrus, the ruler of the synagogue (Mk 5:21ff, 35–43).
- No. 30: Lazarus in Bethany (Jn 11:1–45).

Chapter 3
The Meaning of Miracles

3.1 What Is a Miracle?

What is a miracle? Not all people understand the same thing by the term miracle. In common parlance, a miracle is an "extraordinary event that contradicts the laws of nature or all experience and is therefore attributed to the direct influence of a divine power or supernatural forces, or an event that arouses astonishment".[1]

Whether something is seen as a miracle or not, however, also depends to a large extent on the attitude of the observer. Here are a few examples[2]:

- According to D. Hume, a miracle is a violation of natural laws.
- According to the religious view, a miracle is an extraordinary event that can be attributed to the intervention of God.
- According to the agnostic view, a miracle is an extraordinary law of nature.

No uniform definition can be found among theologians. Only divine intervention is common to all theological definitions of the term miracle. Another common feature for the perception of a miracle is the rare occurrence of the phenomenon in question.

3.2 Is There Still Belief in Miracles Today?

Experiences of miracles are still widespread. Every second German believes in miracles. This was the conclusion of the Allensbach Institute, which conducted a survey on the subject of "miracles" on behalf of the Frankfurter Allgemeine Zeitung.[3] In this

---

[1] Duden - Deutsches Universalwörterbuch, 6. Aufl. Mannheim 2006 [CD-ROM].

[2] Wunder. (2014, December 04). Retrieved from https://www.spektrum.de/lexikon/psychologie/wunder/17003.

[3] FAZ vom 20.09.2006: Wer glaubt an Wunder, von Professor Elisabeth Noelle und Dr. Thomas Petersen.

M. Ledochowski, *The Miracles of the Bible Viewed Differently*,
https://doi.org/10.1007/978-3-031-51639-9_3

survey, fifty-six percent of Germans answered the question "do you believe in miracles?" with "yes". Fifty-four percent of the respondents were convinced that there are cases in which someone senses an impending danger in advance. Fifty-one percent believe in guardian angels, forty-five percent think it is possible to be in mental contact with someone far away. Only thirty percent of Germans think that what many call miracles are, in fact, pure coincidences. It hardly made a difference whether someone had a higher education or not (58% vs. 55%). In the self-employed group, belief in miracles was even more widespread (64%) than, for example, among skilled workers (52%). There was also no significant difference between the generations.[4]

In Iceland, it is said that more than half of the population believes in nature spirits, elves and trolls, and more than ninety percent of the population believes that such beings can exist. Yes, even the Ministry of Construction of Iceland heeds such beliefs and takes into account the "habitat" of elves and other nature spirits when planning roads and buildings. In the past, the Ministry of Construction even employed its own folklorist for this purpose. His job was to look after displaced elf houses. According to Icelanders, elves who are deprived of their place of residence can develop into uncomfortable troublemakers: Bulldozers suddenly stop working, or there are frequent accidents on the construction site.[5]

There is a lot of money to be made from belief in miracles. The non-clerical esoteric industry in Germany alone has an estimated annual turnover of 25 billion euros, writes S. Seiderer in an article in "Die Welt" on the occasion of the 25th anniversary of the esoteric fair.[6] The church institutions also own quite a lot of assets. In an article by Focus Online, the total financial assets of the Catholic Church in Germany are estimated at 150 billion euros. In an article in the Frankfurter Allgemeine Zeitung, the author estimates the annual church income at 5.2 billion euros for the Catholic Church and 4.62 billion euros for the Protestant Church.[7] However, the assets of other religious communities are likely to be similar, depending on their numbers.

Whether these figures are correct or not, they show that people are willing to pay for belief in the afterlife, belief in miracles and belief in something "incomprehensible". Obviously, an important need of people is being satisfied here, otherwise they would not spend so much money on it. And it doesn't seem to matter whether it is established religions or esotericism. What seems to be important above all is the belief in the otherworldly. One does not risk being socially isolated if one professes belief in miracles in public. It seems that it is rather the other way round. Those who do not believe in miracles find little understanding for their view among the population.

---

[4] FAZ vom ? 20.09.2006FAZ Wer glaubt an Wunder, von Professor Elisabeth Noelle und Dr. Thomas Petersen.

[5] http://www.geo.de/GEOlino/kreativ/island-insel-der-elfen-und-trolle-2566.html (Abruf am 25.1.2015).

[6] Sophia Seiderer, Mit Esoterik lässt sich reales Geld machen, Die Welt vom 16.04.2011.

[7] Ralph Bollman: Wie reich Deutschlands Kirchen wirklich sind. Frankfurter Allgemeine vom 20.10.2013.

Why does the belief in miracles persist for such a long time, not only among the laity, but also among theologians? It is a well-known phenomenon that new findings are often rejected. In scientific circles this is also called the Semmelweis effect, named after the Austro-Hungarian doctor P. Semmelweis (1818–1865), who was the first to recognize that disinfecting hands could significantly reduce the mortality of mothers from childbed fever. He is therefore also regarded as the "saviour of mothers" because his findings spared thousands of mothers from death through childbed fever. In his time, he met with fierce resistance from his doctor colleagues, who accused him of speculation. Resistance by "experts" against new knowledge that makes familiar behaviour look questionable is called the Semmelweis effect because of this history. The tendency to reject dissenting opinions and to marginalize those who hold them seems to be in the nature of man; this is true even for science.[8] This may also explain why a different interpretation of biblical miracles has been rejected by theologians for centuries.

3.3 Why Do so Many People Believe in Miracles?

The belief in miracles is a part of religious faith itself. This explains why religious people in particular are more likely to believe in miracles than agnostics. "The miracle is faith's favourite child", Goethe already wrote in Doctor Faust. In addition, there is something comforting about belief in miracles. Miracle stories help us to understand the world where there seem to be no explanations for us. For most people, miracles represent something good, beautiful or saving. When nothing else helps, people hope for a miracle. In hopeless situations, only a miracle can help. This is also the case with people in the terminal stage of an illness.[9] We seek security in the divine, the supernatural or through spiritual beings.[10] People who feel threatened in their existence are more likely to believe in miracles, a social psychological study has found. The study analysed data from 15,400 people surveyed in 16 countries in Latin America. The following was found[11]:

- That there is a positive correlation between miracle experiences and financial insecurity (poor people are more likely to experience miracles than rich people).

[8] Gerhard Medicus: Was uns Menschen verbindet. Angebote zur Verständigung zwischen Natur- Kultur- und Geisteswissenschaften. 6. erweiterte Auflage, VWB-Verlag für Wissenschaft und Bildung, Berlin 2022. Internetlink: https://doi.org/10.25651/1.2022.0001.

[9] Paiva CE. When the belief in a miracle is the last thread of hope. Palliat Support Care. 2013 Oct;11(5):443–4. doi: https://doi.org/10.1017/S1478951512000302. Epub 2012 Jul 30. PMID: 22840235.

[10] FAZ vom ? 20.09.2006FAZ Wer glaubt an Wunder, von Professor Elisabeth Noelle und Dr. Thomas Petersen.

[11] Eschler, E. (2020). In the Valley of the Shadow of Death: Insecurity and Miraculous Experiences. Review of Religious Research, 62(3). doi: https://doi.org/10.1007/s13644-020-00419-w.

- That the wealthy and well-educated are more likely to experience miracles when their lives become uncertain or threatened (people who have fallen in status are more likely to experience miracles than people who have been favoured by fate).
- That more Protestants than Catholics believed they had experienced a divine apparition.

The belief in miracles has something comforting for all people who no longer know how to help themselves. As I said, in a hopeless situation, only a miracle can promise salvation. And no one wants to miss this belief in salvation. No matter how rich or educated someone may be, most people get into a (seemingly) hopeless situation at some point. At the latest, at the time of death, it concerns every human being to come to terms with this hopelessness. Belief in a religion and belief in miracles helps one at this point at the latest. This may be one reason why no one wants to be deprived of their faith in the supernatural and their belief in miracles.

3.4 How Does Religiosity and Belief in Miracles Come About in the First Place?

Belief in miracles and belief in God are often connected. While belief in miracles primarily promises comfort in hopeless situations, the matter is somewhat more complex in the case of belief in God and religiosity. Neurotheology deals with the phenomenon of religiosity and belief in miracles in a scientific sense. This still relatively young branch of science investigates the relationship between the body and religious experiences; experiences such as changes during meditation, near-death experiences, trance states, feelings such as "being at one with the universe", encounters with supernatural beings, etc. Neurotheology tries to clarify whether these experiences are imaginary or real: what processes occur in the brain during such experiences; whether such experiences cause changes in the brain, or whether the brain creates such experiences. Neurotheologists also look for the seat of religiosity in the brain—whether there is also a centre of religious experience in the brain analogous to a language centre, vision centre, hearing centre, etc. Or whether there are changes in the metabolism of neurotransmitters. Whether the EEG changes in situations of religious experience, or whether there are differences in the genetic make-up of believers and non-believers.

Until recently, neurotheology had a difficult time being recognized by the scientific community. A brief summary of the results of neurotheological research to date is given here:

3.4.1 Neurotransmitters and Religiousness

Serotonin: Hallucinogens have been used to induce spiritual experiences since ancient times.[12] Most of them act on the serotonergic system. Especially; substances with effects on the 5-HT1A receptor can be associated with spiritual experiences. Substances such as LSD or psilocybin can even trigger spiritual experiences, mystical experiences and feelings of ecstasy.

Dopamine: Dopamine seems to play a role in the development of feelings of religiosity. Drugs with a dopamine agonist effect can increase religious feelings, those with a dopamine antagonist effect can cause religious experiences to disappear. Thus, patients with Parkinson's Disease also show less interest in religion and consistently have lower scores on measures of religiosity than control subjects. Prefrontal dopaminergic networks could support the motivational aspects of religiosity.[13]

Oxytocin: Oxytocin is often called the "cuddle hormone" because it is crucial for social bonding. For example, oxytocin is produced more frequently during breastfeeding and not only causes breast milk to flow, but also triggers a more intimate bond between the mother and the child. Oxytocin also plays an important role during orgasm and leads to increased bonding between sexual partners. Oxytocin can also have an effect on spirituality. Oxytocin seems to increase the feeling of connection with a higher power or the world. If people are given oxytocin in the form of a nasal spray before meditation, the spiritual experience is intensified. This effect is maintained for several days.[14]

Neuropeptide Y (NPY): In a study of young adults, a positive correlation was found between serum neuropeptide Y levels and religious commitment. This could be an indicator that neuropeptide Y is a biological correlate of religious commitment.[15]

---

[12] Doblin RE, Christiansen M, Jerome L, Burge B. The Past and Future of Psychedelic Science: An Introduction to This Issue. J Psychoactive Drugs. 2019 Apr–Jun;51(2):93–97. doi: https://doi.org/10.1080/02791072.2019.1606472. PMID: 31132970.

[13] McNamara P, Durso R, Brown A. Religiosity in patients with Parkinson's disease. Neuropsychiatr Dis Treat. 2006 Sep;2(3):341–8. doi: https://doi.org/10.2147/nedt.2006.2.3.341. PMID: 19412480; PMCID: PMC2671825.

[14] Van Cappellen P, Way BM, Isgett SF, Fredrickson BL. Effects of oxytocin administration on spirituality and emotional responses to meditation. Soc Cogn Affect Neurosci. 2016 Oct;11(10):1579–87. doi: https://doi.org/10.1093/scan/nsw078. Epub 2016 Jun 17. PMID: 27317929; PMCID: PMC5040919.

[15] Tønnesen, M. T., Miani, A., Pedersen, A. S., Mitkidis, P., Zak, P. J., & Winterdahl, M. (2019). Neuropeptide Y and religious commitment in healthy young women. Acta Neuropsychiatr., 31(2), 106–112. doi: https://doi.org/10.1017/neu.2018.34.

Placebo effect: A basic spiritual attitude also seems to have an influence on the effect of placebos.[16] So one can well imagine that those people who believed in Jesus and his disciples were more likely to be eligible for miraculous healings.

3.4.2 *Genetics and Religiousness*

Genospirituality is the name of the controversial field that studies the relationship between spiritual and religious behaviour and individual genes.[17] Some polymorphisms of the dopamine D4 receptor (DRD4 polymorphisms) tend to be associated with increased pro-social (religious) actions and increased religious feelings.[18] In his book "The God Gene: How Faith is Hardwired into our Genes",[19] D. Hamer argues that a variation in the VMAT2 gene plays a role in the propensity for spiritual experiences. Another study found a link between religiosity and 5-HTTLPR and AP-2beta genotypes.[20] Overall, however, the influence of genetic polymorphisms seems to be limited.[21]

3.4.3 *Epilepsy and Religiousness*

Epilepsy was already associated with behavioural changes and religious zeal by Hippocrates. Since that time, it was believed that the seizures were due to demonic or divine influences (Morbus sacer). Some scientists believe that the visions and spiritual experiences of famous prophets, including Ezekiel, Buddha, Mohammed, and Joan

---

[16] Kohls N, Sauer S, Offenbächer M, Giordano J. Spirituality: an overlooked predictor of placebo effects? Philos Trans R Soc Lond B Biol Sci. 2011 Jun 27;366(1572):1838–48. doi: https://doi.org/10.1098/rstb.2010.0389. PMID: 21576141; PMCID: PMC3130399.

[17] Blum K, Thompson B, Oscar-Berman M, Giordano J, Braverman E, Femino J, Barh D, Downs W, Smpatico T, Schoenthaler S. Genospirituality: Our Beliefs, Our Genomes, and Addictions. J Addict Res Ther. 2013 Oct 10;5(4):162. doi: https://doi.org/10.4172/2155-6105.1000162.1000162. PMID: 24971227; PMCID: PMC4068016.

[18] Sasaki JY, Kim HS, Mojaverian T, Kelley LD, Park IY, Janusonis S. Religion priming differentially increases prosocial behavior among variants of the dopamine D4 receptor (DRD4) gene. Soc Cogn Affect Neurosci. 2013 Feb;8(2):209–15. doi: https://doi.org/10.1093/scan/nsr089. Epub 2011 Dec 23. PMID: 22198971; PMCID: PMC3575725.

[19] Dean H. Hamer; The God Gene: How Faith Is Hardwired into Our Genes; Knopf Doubleday Publishing Group ISBN 978-0-307-27693-3.

[20] Nilsson KW, Damberg M, Ohrvik J, Leppert J, Lindström L, Anckarsäter H, Oreland L. Genes encoding for AP-2beta and the Serotonin Transporter are associated with the Personality Character Spiritual Acceptance. Neurosci Lett. 2007 Jan 16;411(3):233-7. doi: https://doi.org/10.1016/j.neulet.2006.10.051. Epub 2006 Nov 22. PMID: 17123722.

[21] Laje G, Perlis RH, Rush AJ, McMahon FJ. Pharmacogenetics studies in STAR*D: strengths, limitations, and results. Psychiatr Serv. 2009 Nov;60(11):1446–57. doi: https://doi.org/10.1176/appi.ps.60.11.1446. PMID: 19880459; PMCID: PMC3775610.

of Arc, were actually of epileptic origin.[22] Patients with temporal lobe epilepsy sometimes have religious experiences during seizures.[23] Personality changes in the sense of hyper-religiousness were also observed between such seizures.[24,25] The conversion of St. Paul and the ecstatic experiences that accompanied it are also associated with seizures in the context of temporal lobe epilepsy.[26] In any case, there is much evidence that epilepsy, especially when it comes to temporal lobe seizures, is associated with religious feelings and hyper-religious behaviour.

3.4.4 Psychiatric Disorders and Spirituality

Religious beliefs and practices have long been associated with hysteria, neurosis and psychotic delusions. However, recent studies have shown that religiosity or spirituality can serve as a psychological and social resource for coping with stress.[27] Religion and spirituality thus have the capacity to promote or impair mental health.[28]

3.4.5 Neuroanatomical Variability, Brain Lesions and Religiosity

When people have to undergo surgery as part of a brain tumour treatment or suffer a failure of certain parts of the brain due to a stroke, this can be accompanied by personality changes. Based on these changes, conclusions can be drawn about the functionality of these sections of the brain. Likewise, anatomical differences in religious and non-religious people can be used to draw conclusions about the functions

[22] Devinsky O, Lai G. Spirituality and religion in epilepsy. Epilepsy Behav. 2008 May;12(4):636–43. doi: https://doi.org/10.1016/j.yebeh.2007.11.011. Epub 2008 Jan 2. PMID: 18171635.

[23] Ogata A, Miyakawa T. Religious experiences in epileptic patients with a focus on ictus-related episodes. Psychiatry Clin Neurosci. 1998 Jun;52(3):321–5. doi: https://doi.org/10.1046/j.1440-1819.1998.00397.x. PMID: 9681585.

[24] Devinsky J, Schachter S. Norman Geschwind's contribution to the understanding of behavioral changes in temporal lobe epilepsy: the February 1974 lecture. Epilepsy Behav. 2009 Aug;15(4):417–24. doi: https://doi.org/10.1016/j.yebeh.2009.06.006. Epub 2009 Jul 29. PMID: 19640791.

[25] Garcia-Santibanez R, Sarva H. Isolated Hyperreligiosity in a Patient with Temporal Lobe Epilepsy. Case Rep Neurol Med. 2015;2015:235856. doi: https://doi.org/10.1155/2015/235856. Epub 2015 Aug 13. PMID: 26351599; PMCID: PMC4550801.

[26] Landsborough D. St Paul and temporal lobe epilepsy. J Neurol Neurosurg Psychiatry. 1987 Jun;50(6):659–64. doi: https://doi.org/10.1136/jnnp.50.6.659. PMID: 3302109; PMCID: PMC1032067.

[27] Koenig HG. Research on religion, spirituality, and mental health: a review. Can J Psychiatry. 2009 May;54(5):283–91. doi: https://doi.org/10.1177/070674370905400502. PMID: 19497160.

[28] Weber SR, Pargament KI. The role of religion and spirituality in mental health. Curr Opin Psychiatry. 2014 Sep;27(5):358–63. doi: https://doi.org/10.1097/YCO.0000000000000080. PMID: 25046080.

of certain areas of the brain. For example, differences in religious and non-religious people could be found in MRI examinations. In people who described themselves as very religious, an increased volume was found in the right temporal cortex (BA21) and a decreased volume in the left orbitofrontal cortex (BA11). People with doubts about the existence of God showed an increased volume of the right precuneus.[29]

Magical thinking could be found more often in people with injuries in the prefrontal cortex.[30] Increased feelings of religiosity and spirituality could be found after lesions of the periaqueductal grey matter in the anterior brainstem (midbrain) whereas,[31] in contrast, another study found no structural differences in the brains of religious people compared to non-religious people.[32]

3.4.6 *Blood Flow and Metabolic Changes in the Brain and Religiosity*

Positron emission tomography (PET) can be used to examine the metabolic activity of individual brain sections, and functional magnetic resonance imaging (fMRI) can be used to examine the blood flow to individual brain areas. Here, too, there are studies that found differences in religious and non-religious people.[33] PET studies with isotopes directed against serotonin receptors showed increased activity in the median raphe nucleus in individuals with spiritual experiences.[34] There are numerous studies that have demonstrated differences in anatomy, functions, and metabolism

[29] Kapogiannis D, Barbey AK, Su M, Krueger F, Grafman J. Neuroanatomical variability of religiosity. PLoS One. 2009 Sep 28;4(9):e7180. doi: https://doi.org/10.1371/journal.pone.0007180. PMID: 19784372; PMCID: PMC2746321.

[30] Zhong W, Krueger F, Wilson M, Bulbulia J, Grafman J. Prefrontal brain lesions reveal magical ideation arises from enhanced religious experiences. Peace Confl. 2018 May;24(2):245–249. doi: https://doi.org/10.1037/pac0000336. PMID: 30364497; PMCID: PMC6197485.

[31] Ferguson MA, Schaper FLWVJ, Cohen A, Siddiqi S, Merrill SM, Nielsen JA, Grafman J, Urgesi C, Fabbro F, Fox MD. A Neural Circuit for Spirituality and Religiosity Derived From Patients With Brain Lesions. Biol Psychiatry. 2022 Feb 15;91(4):380–388. doi: https://doi.org/10.1016/j.biopsych.2021.06.016. Epub 2021 Jun 29. PMID: 34454698; PMCID: PMC8714871.

[32] van Elk M, Snoek L. The relationship between individual differences in gray matter volume and religiosity and mystical experiences: A preregistered voxel-based morphometry study. Eur J Neurosci. 2020 Feb;51(3):850–865. doi: https://doi.org/10.1111/ejn.14563. Epub 2019 Sep 23. PMID: 31465601; PMCID: PMC7079225.

[33] Rim JI, Ojeda JC, Svob C, Kayser J, Drews E, Kim Y, Tenke CE, Skipper J, Weissman MM. Current Understanding of Religion, Spirituality, and Their Neurobiological Correlates. Harv Rev Psychiatry. 2019 Sep/Oct;27(5):303–316. doi: https://doi.org/10.1097/HRP.0000000000000232. PMID: 31490186; PMCID: PMC7195862.

[34] Kim JH, Son YD, Kim JH, Choi EJ, Lee SY, Joo YH, Kim YB, Cho ZH. Self-transcendence trait and its relationship with in vivo serotonin transporter availability in brainstem raphe nuclei: An ultra-high resolution PET-MRI study. Brain Res. 2015 Dec 10;1629:63–71. doi: https://doi.org/10.1016/j.brainres.2015.10.006. Epub 2015 Oct 13. PMID: 26459992.

in the brains of people. For an overview of the neurobiology of spirituality, see E. Mohandas.[35]

When studying religiosity and trying to assign it to different brain regions, one comes to the view that, strictly speaking, there are different functions involved. One can distinguish three different types of subjectively felt religiosity, which can also be assigned to different brain regions:

1. Magical thinking (the unshakeable belief in connections, even if these do not exist objectively).
2. Spirituality (the feeling of being one with the universe or having intense experiences of God).
3. Belief in God or something divine (religiosity in the narrower sense).

3.4.6.1 Magical Thinking

In psychology, **magical thinking** is a type of thinking in which a person assumes that their thoughts, words, or actions have an influence on causally unrelated events. Conventional rules of cause and effect are ignored. In anthropology, magical thinking stands for ideas that deal with supernatural powers and express themselves in rituals.

In childhood, magical thinking can be seen as part of the animistic-magical developmental phase of the two to five-year-old child. Before a child develops rational thinking, magical thinking occurs, for example, in the form of belief in the effects of magic, incantations or wishful thinking. In adulthood, magical thinking can be part of several attenuated psychotic symptoms, but not all magical thinking is psychotic.

Examples of magical thinking are

- There are supernatural remote effects (remote healings in the Bible).
- Objects can transfer properties of their owners (voodoo magic).
- Things that have a property in common are also similar in others (cf. homeopathy, the doctrine of signatures or analogy magic).
- One can influence the outside world through words, formulas, spells or mere thoughts (prayers, rituals, exorcisms etc.).
- The future is foreseeable, certain things or processes have a foreshadowing (omen).
- Symbols, for example amulets, would have an effect (belief in angels, voodoo etc.).
- Certain people would have supernatural powers or could force beings with such powers into their service.
- Spirits, gods, or secret societies can link events or phenomena that are separate from each other.

[35] Mohandas E. Neurobiology of spirituality. Mens Sana Monogr. 2008 Jan;6(1):63–80. doi: https://doi.org/10.4103/0973-1229.33001. PMID: 22013351; PMCID: PMC3190564.

3.4.6.2 Spirituality

Spirituality is defined as the search for and turning towards a transcendent reality, which cannot be grasped by the senses and cannot be explained rationally, and which underlies the material world.[36] Spiritual insights can be connected with questions of meaning of existence, with the experience of the wholeness of the world in its connectedness with one's own existence, with the "ultimate highest truth" in one's own life. It is not a matter of mental insights, or communication about them. But in each case it is a matter of intense, highly personal experiences that have a direct impact on the way of life and the ethical ideas of the person. A religious conviction is a prerequisite, but it does not have to be associated with a particular religion. There is no generally accepted definition of the term. In Christianity, the term spirituality is used synonymously with piety.

3.4.6.3 Religiosity

Religiosity is the term used to describe piety.[37] On Wikipedia, one finds a 125-word, rather confusing definition that tries not to leave out, any aspect of religiosity.[38] I would like to refer to religiosity as belief in something higher, in distinction to spirituality and magical thinking. Regardless of whether it is a belief in one God (monotheism), in several Gods (polytheism), in angels, demons, invisible beings (spiritualism) or other beings. This is usually accompanied by a fervent desire for salvation and a belief in a further life after death. I would rather assign the heartfelt desire for enlightenment to spirituality, whereby religiosity and spirituality often go hand in hand. If religiosity is associated with anxiety or stress, this can have negative effects on health. This is called "neurotic religiosity".[39] People's religiosity can be divided into two types according to the nature of their motivation:[40]

- Intrinsic religiosity: people who align and satisfy their needs according to their religious beliefs (goal of religious doctrine).
- Extrinsic religiosity: people for whom there are personal benefits in belonging to a religious community, e.g. as a distraction, justification or for status reasons (contradiction to religious doctrine, see also hypocrisy).

---

[36] Autoren der Wikimedia-Projekte. (2003, July 09). Spiritualität—Wikipedia. Retrieved from https://de.wikipedia.org/w/index.php?title=Spiritualit%C3%A4t&oldid=225235861.

[37] Duden, Deutsches Universalwörterbuch, 6. Auflage, Mannheim 2006 (CD-ROM).

[38] Autoren der Wikimedia-Projekte. (2005, July 12). Religiosität—Wikipedia. Retrieved from https://de.wikipedia.org/w/index.php?title=Religiosit%C3%A4t&oldid=224302469.

[39] Werner Stangl: Stichwort *„Religionspsychologie" im Online Lexikon für Psychologie und Pädagogik*. Online Lexikon für Psychologie und Pädagogik.

[40] Ursula Eder: *Religiosität als Selbstaufwertung: Eine Metaanalyse der Beziehung zwischen sozial erwünschten Antworten und Religiosität*, Teil der Seminararbeit *Zur Psychologie der Religion*, Universität Wien 2011.

The various psychological aspects of religion, spirituality and magical thinking are dealt with by the psychology of religion, which is seen as a sub-field of applied psychology.[41]

[41] Religionspsychologie. Online Lexikon für Psychologie und Pädagogik. (2022, August 22).

Epilogue

When miracles of the Bible are seen through the eyes of a doctor, the aim is not to destroy religious feelings or faith. On the contrary, as human beings, we all carry within us the predisposition for religiosity. Just as there is hunger, thirst, desire for love and recognition, well-being, and the search for many kinds of reward, there is also the pursuit of religiosity and spirituality. If neuroscience is to be believed, these feelings can be found in brain regions that are developmentally old brain regions, that also play an important role in our social behaviour. In any case, religion makes sense from the point of view of evolution and is also likely to improve the ability of individuals to survive in a group.

In addition, religion has other functions

- For many people, it provides comfort. After all, we are all born with a death sentence. We sit on "death row" all our lives, so to speak, waiting for execution without knowing when and how death will befall us. Actually, a terrible idea, which is hardly to be borne by some people. Belief in a God and an afterlife can offer help here.
- For many people, religion offers a way to find meaning in their lives. Religion represents a sort of "logotherapy" in the psychotherapeutic sense.[1]
- With the view of an afterlife, religion offers many people a chance of compensatory justice for all the injustice and suffering they have experienced during their lives. Whether this is really so, no one can determine. But in any case, these are comforting thoughts.
- After all, many religions offer guidelines for an ethically moral life, a prerequisite for living together peacefully.
- In sum, religions have a social and psycho-hygienic function.

Religious institutions often feel they are the guardians of moral guidelines. In this way, they gain enormous influence on people and gain power over them. However,

[1] Frankl VE. Logotherapy. Isr Ann Psychiatr Relat Discip. 1967;5(2):142–55. PMID: 5247330.

M. Ledochowski, *The Miracles of the Bible Viewed Differently*,
https://doi.org/10.1007/978-3-031-51639-9

this was not always exercised for the benefit of the people. In the last few years, more and more people are therefore "converting" to atheism or calling themselves agnostics. They leave their religious institution because they no longer find there what they were actually looking for.

It is astonishing that atheists often already see themselves as acting more morally or ethically than followers of many religions. A reason for it might lie in the fact that these people recognized that they actually do themselves a favour by their high-quality moral thinking and acting. This is not a plea for all people to become do-gooders, but to recognize that ethical moral thinking and acting serves one's own reward system and thus makes one happy. Every human being carries, in the sense of Kant, "his categorical imperative" in himself[2]—a conscience that tells him at any time what is okay and what is not. If a person follows this conscience, his brain is built in such a way that it rewards itself for doing so. We know today that not only a healthy lifestyle, but also a "calm and clear conscience" leads to a much better quality of life. It pays off therefore from purely egoistic motives to live morally, following one's conscience, be it as an atheist or as a member of a religion, as long as one feels comfortable in it.

---

[2] Pleger, W. (2017). Der kategorische Imperativ (Kant). Das gute Leben. J.B. Metzler. doi: https://doi.org/10.1007/978-3-476-04483-9_12.

SPRINGER NATURE

GPSR Compliance

The European Union's (EU) General Product Safety Regulation (GPSR) is a set of rules that requires consumer products to be safe and our obligations to ensure this.

If you have any concerns about our products, you can contact us on ProductSafety@springernature.com

In case Publisher is established outside the EU, the EU authorized representative is:

Springer Nature Customer Service Center GmbH
Europaplatz 3
69115 Heidelberg, Germany

The manufacturer's authorised representative in the EU is Springer Nature Customer Service Centre GmbH, Europaplatz 3, 69115 Heidelberg, Germany. If you have any concerns regarding our products, please contact ProductSafety@springernature.com

Printed and bound by CPI Group (UK) Ltd, Croydon, CR0 4YY
01/10/2026
02225876-0014